Hearing Loss and Healthy Aging

WORKSHOP SUMMARY

D1530793

Tracy A. Lustig and Steve Olson, *Rapporteurs*

Forum on Aging, Disability, and Independence

Board on Health Sciences Policy

Division of Behavioral and Social Sciences and Education

INSTITUTE OF MEDICINE *AND*
NATIONAL RESEARCH COUNCIL
OF THE NATIONAL ACADEMIES

THE NATIONAL ACADEMIES PRESS
Washington, D.C.
www.nap.edu

THE NATIONAL ACADEMIES PRESS   500 Fifth Street, NW   Washington, DC 20001

This activity was supported by contracts between the National Academy of Sciences and the Academy of Doctors of Audiology; the American Academy of Audiology; the American Academy of Otolaryngology–Head and Neck Surgery; American Geriatrics Society; the American Speech-Language-Hearing Association; Cochlear Americas; the European Hearing Instrument Manufacturers Association; the Gerontological Society of America; the Hearing Industries Association; the Hearing Loss Association of America; Hi HealthInnovations; LeadingAge; MED-EL Corporation, USA; the National Institute on Aging (Contract No. HHSN26300038); the National Institutes of Health's National Institute on Aging and National Institute on Deafness and Other Communication Disorders (Contract No. HHSN26300048); The SCAN Foundation (Contract No. 12-004), Sound World Solutions; United HealthCare; the U.S. Department of Education's National Institute on Disability and Rehabilitation Research (Contract No. ED-OSE-12-P-0066); and the U.S. Department of Veterans Affairs (Contract No. VA268-12-P-0014). The views presented in this publication do not necessarily reflect the views of the organizations or agencies that provided support for the activity.

International Standard Book Number-13:   978-0-309-30226-5
International Standard Book Number-10:   0-309-30226-9

Additional copies of this workshop summary are available for sale from the National Academies Press, 500 Fifth Street, NW, Keck 360, Washington, DC 20001; (800) 624-6242 or (202) 334-3313; http://www.nap.edu.

For more information about the Institute of Medicine, visit the IOM home page at: **www.iom.edu.**

Printed in the United States of America

The serpent has been a symbol of long life, healing, and knowledge among almost all cultures and religions since the beginning of recorded history. The serpent adopted as a logotype by the Institute of Medicine is a relief carving from ancient Greece, now held by the Staatliche Museen in Berlin.

Suggested citation: IOM (Institute of Medicine) and NRC (National Research Council). 2014. *Hearing loss and healthy aging: Workshop summary.* Washington, DC: The National Academies Press.

THE NATIONAL ACADEMIES
Advisers to the Nation on Science, Engineering, and Medicine

The **National Academy of Sciences** is a private, nonprofit, self-perpetuating society of distinguished scholars engaged in scientific and engineering research, dedicated to the furtherance of science and technology and to their use for the general welfare. Upon the authority of the charter granted to it by the Congress in 1863, the Academy has a mandate that requires it to advise the federal government on scientific and technical matters. Dr. Ralph J. Cicerone is president of the National Academy of Sciences.

The **National Academy of Engineering** was established in 1964, under the charter of the National Academy of Sciences, as a parallel organization of outstanding engineers. It is autonomous in its administration and in the selection of its members, sharing with the National Academy of Sciences the responsibility for advising the federal government. The National Academy of Engineering also sponsors engineering programs aimed at meeting national needs, encourages education and research, and recognizes the superior achievements of engineers. Dr. C. D. Mote, Jr., is president of the National Academy of Engineering.

The **Institute of Medicine** was established in 1970 by the National Academy of Sciences to secure the services of eminent members of appropriate professions in the examination of policy matters pertaining to the health of the public. The Institute acts under the responsibility given to the National Academy of Sciences by its congressional charter to be an adviser to the federal government and, upon its own initiative, to identify issues of medical care, research, and education. Dr. Harvey V. Fineberg is president of the Institute of Medicine.

The **National Research Council** was organized by the National Academy of Sciences in 1916 to associate the broad community of science and technology with the Academy's purposes of furthering knowledge and advising the federal government. Functioning in accordance with general policies determined by the Academy, the Council has become the principal operating agency of both the National Academy of Sciences and the National Academy of Engineering in providing services to the government, the public, and the scientific and engineering communities. The Council is administered jointly by both Academies and the Institute of Medicine. Dr. Ralph J. Cicerone and Dr. C. D. Mote, Jr., are chair and vice chair, respectively, of the National Research Council.

www.national-academies.org

PLANNING COMMITTEE FOR A WORKSHOP ON HEARING LOSS AND HEALTHY AGING[1]

ALAN M. JETTE (*Co-Chair*), Professor of Health Policy and Management and Director, Health and Disability Research Institute, Boston University School of Public Health

FRANK R. LIN (*Co-Chair*), Assistant Professor of Otolaryngology–Head and Neck Surgery, Geriatric Medicine, Mental Health, and Epidemiology, Johns Hopkins University

BRENDA BATTAT, Executive Director (retired), Hearing Loss Association of America

LUCILLE B. BECK, National Program Director, Audiology and Speech Pathology, and Chief Consultant, Rehabilitation and Prosthetic Services, Patient Care Services, U.S. Department of Veterans Affairs

NIKOLAI BISGAARD, Vice President, Intellectual Property Rights and Industry Relations, GN ReSound A/S

KAREN J. CRUICKSHANKS, Professor of Ophthalmology and Visual Sciences and Population Health Sciences, University of Wisconsin School of Medicine and Public Health

LUIGI FERRUCCI, Scientific Director and Chief, Longitudinal Studies Section, National Institute on Aging

JAMES FIRMAN, President and Chief Executive Officer, National Council on Aging

CAROLE M. ROGIN, President, Hearing Industries Association

---

[1] Institute of Medicine and National Research Council planning committees are solely responsible for organizing the workshop, identifying topics, and choosing speakers. The responsibility for the published workshop summary rests with the workshop rapporteurs and the institution.

FORUM ON AGING, DISABILITY, AND INDEPENDENCE[1]

ALAN M. JETTE (*Co-Chair*), Boston University School of Public Health, MA
JOHN W. ROWE (*Co-Chair*), Columbia University, New York, NY
KELLY BUCKLAND, National Council on Independent Living, Washington, DC
JOE CALDWELL, National Council on Aging, Washington, DC
MARGARET L. CAMPBELL, National Institute on Disability and Rehabilitation Research, Washington, DC
EILEEN M. CRIMMINS, University of Southern California, Los Angeles
PEGGYE DILWORTH-ANDERSON, Gillings School of Global Public Health, University of North Carolina, Chapel Hill
STEVEN C. EDELSTEIN, PHI, Bronx, NY
THOMAS E. EDES, U.S. Department of Veterans Affairs, Washington, DC
TERRY FULMER, Bouvé College of Health Sciences, Northeastern University, Boston, MA
NAOMI L. GERBER, Center for the Study of Chronic Illness and Disability, George Mason University, Fairfax, VA
ROBERT HORNYAK, Administration for Community Living, Washington, DC
LISA I. IEZZONI, Harvard Medical School, Boston, MA
JUDITH D. KASPER, Johns Hopkins Bloomberg School of Public Health, Baltimore, MD
KATHY KREPCIO, John J. Heldrich Center for Workforce Development, Rutgers, The State University of New Jersey, New Brunswick, NJ
NANCY LUNDEBJERG, American Geriatrics Society, New York, NY
RHONDA MEDOWS, United HealthCare, Washington, DC
LARRY MINNIX, LeadingAge, Washington, DC
ARI NE'EMAN, National Council on Disability, Washington, DC
RENÉ SEIDEL, The SCAN Foundation, Long Beach, CA
JACK W. SMITH, U.S. Department of Defense, Falls Church, VA
RICHARD SUZMAN, National Institute on Aging, Bethesda, MD

---

[1] Institute of Medicine and National Research Council forums do not issue, review, or approve individual documents. The responsibility for the published summary rests with the workshop rapporteurs and the institution.

Reviewers

This workshop summary has been reviewed in draft form by individuals chosen for their diverse perspectives and technical expertise, in accordance with procedures approved by the National Research Council's Report Review Committee. The purpose of this independent review is to provide candid and critical comments that will assist the institution in making its published workshop summary as sound as possible and to ensure that the workshop summary meets institutional standards for objectivity, evidence, and responsiveness to the study charge. The review comments and draft manuscript remain confidential to protect the integrity of the process. We wish to thank the following individuals for their review of this workshop summary:

JUDY R. DUBNO, Medical University of South Carolina
NOREEN GIBBENS, Hi HealthInnovations
ELLEN MORGENSTERN, The Foundation of the National
Committee to Preserve Social Security and Medicare

Although the reviewers listed above have provided many constructive comments and suggestions, they did not see the final draft of the workshop summary before its release. The review of this workshop summary was overseen by **DAVID B. REUBEN,** University of California, Los Angeles. Appointed by the Institute of Medicine, he was responsible for making certain that an independent examination of this workshop summary was carried out in accordance with institutional procedures and that all review comments were carefully considered. Responsibility for the final content of this workshop summary rests entirely with the rapporteurs and the institution.

Contents

1

Introduction, Background, and Overview of the Workshop[1]

Being able to communicate is a cornerstone of healthy aging. People need to make themselves understood and to understand others to remain cognitively and socially engaged with families, friends, and other individuals. When they are unable to communicate, people with hearing impairments can become socially isolated, and social isolation can be an important driver of morbidity and mortality in older adults (Cacioppo et al., 2011).

Despite the critical importance of communication, many older adults have hearing loss that interferes with their social interactions and enjoyment of life. This hearing loss is often subtle (Lin, 2012). People may turn up the volume on their televisions or stereos, miss words in a conversation, go to fewer public places where it is difficult to hear, or worry about missing an alarm or notification. In other cases, hearing loss is much more severe, and people may retreat into a hard-to-reach shell. Yet fewer than one in seven older Americans with hearing loss use hearing aids, despite rapidly advancing technologies and innovative approaches to hearing health care (Chien and Lin, 2012). In addition, there may not be an adequate number of professionals trained to address the growing need for hearing health care for older adults. Further, Medicare does not cover "routine hearing exams,

---

[1] The planning committee's role was limited to planning the workshop, and the workshop summary has been prepared by the workshop rapporteurs as a factual summary of what occurred at the workshop. Statements, recommendations, and opinions expressed are those of individual presenters and participants, and are not necessarily endorsed or verified by the Institute of Medicine or the National Research Council, and they should not be construed as reflecting any group consensus.

BOX 1-1
Statement of Task

An ad hoc planning committee will plan and conduct a 2-day public workshop to examine the ways in which age-related hearing loss affects healthy aging, and how the spectrum of public and private stakeholders can work together to address hearing loss in older adults as a public health issue. The workshop will feature invited presentations and discussions that will:

- Describe and characterize the public health significance of hearing loss and the relationship between hearing loss and healthy aging (e.g., medical comorbidities);
- Examine and explore current and future areas of research on hearing loss and healthy aging;
- Discuss comprehensive hearing rehabilitative strategies, including innovative models of care;
- Explore innovative hearing technologies, as well as barriers to their development and use; and
- Consider and discuss short- and long-term collaborative strategies, including public-private partnerships, for approaching age-related hearing loss as a public health priority, for example, developing preventive intervention strategies; improving public awareness; and enhancing professional education.

---

hearing aids, or exams for fitting hearing aids" (CMS, 2014), which can be prohibitively expensive for many older adults.

The Forum on Aging, Disability, and Independence[2] was created by the Institute of Medicine (IOM) in collaboration with the National Research Council (NRC) in 2012 to provide an ongoing, neutral venue where stakeholders in government, academia, industry, foundations, and consumer groups can come together to discuss issues at the intersection of aging and disability. On January 13–14, 2014, the forum held a workshop on age-related hearing loss that brought together more than one hundred researchers, advocates, policy makers, entrepreneurs, regulators, and others to discuss this pressing social and public health issue. The statement of task for the workshop is listed in Box 1-1. A webcast of the workshop is also available.[3]

---

[2] See www.iom.edu/ADIForum (accessed February 24, 2014).
[3] See http://www.iom.edu/Activities/PublicHealth/HearingLossAging/2014-JAN-13.aspx (accessed February 25, 2014).

BACKGROUND

Frank R. Lin
Johns Hopkins University

In the initial session of the workshop, workshop planning committee co-chair Frank Lin, assistant professor of otolaryngology, geriatric medicine, mental health, and epidemiology at the Johns Hopkins University School of Medicine and the Bloomberg School of Public Health, provided background information on age-related hearing loss in the United States and around the world. The prevalence of hearing loss essentially doubles with each decade of age (see Figure 1-1). As a result, nearly two of three Americans ages 70 and above have a clinically meaningful hearing impairment.

The use of hearing aids, in contrast, is "phenomenally low," said Lin (see Figure 1-2). Only about 15 percent of people with a hearing impairment in the United States use a hearing aid. Lin noted that the rate is only a little higher in England and Wales (about 17 percent) even though hearing aids are fully covered by national health insurance there. Furthermore, the prevalence of hearing aid use has not changed substantially for decades in the United States or around the world, Lin said.

A fundamental paradox surrounds hearing loss and the use of hearing

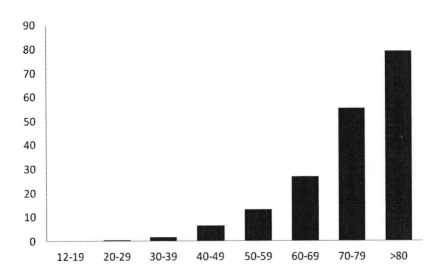

FIGURE 1-1 Prevalence percentage of bilateral hearing loss in the United States by age.
SOURCE: Data from Lin et al., 2011a.

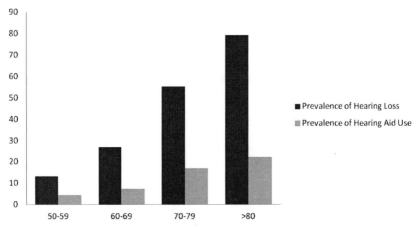

FIGURE 1-2 Prevalence percentage of hearing loss and hearing aid use in the United States by age.
SOURCE: Data from Chien and Lin, 2012.

aids, Lin pointed out. A hearing impairment that would be treated as a serious health issue in a 12-year-old boy is typically met with a shrug in a 72-year-old man. Yet both have a need to communicate with friends, family members, and others to function well in society.

Hearing depends on two basic processes: the peripheral transduction of sound by the cochlea and the central processing or decoding of sound by the brain. Auditory functioning can be measured at multiple levels and in multiple ways, including otoacoustic emissions testing; pure tone audiometry; speech discrimination scores; central auditory measures such as speech in noise and dichotic listening; and subjective hearing and communicative function. These different measures depend both on peripheral inputs or bottom-up processing and on central processing or top-down processing.

Hearing loss often reflects impairments in cochlear functioning that can be assessed with audiometry. For example, an audiogram can be used to calculate the pure-tone average hearing level in decibels (dB) at mid-level frequencies. The cochlea is made up of many cells that cannot regenerate and over time can be damaged by aging, noise, medicines, or other factors. Damage to the cochlea can lead not only to decreased hearing sensitivity but also to poor frequency and temporal encoding of sound. Instead of sending a crisply encoded signal to the brain, the cochlea produces a garbled signal. As Lin described it, people tend to say, "It isn't that I can't hear you. It's that I can't understand you. It sounds like you are mumbling at me all the time." People can still hear what someone is saying if they make an effort, but they have to concentrate much harder to make out what is being said.

Hearing deficits can be associated with other forms of physical and cognitive decline, Lin observed. A fundamental question that remains unanswered is whether and how hearing loss is related to these other negative health outcomes. Do they have common causes in pathological processes, or is hearing loss a modifiable risk factor of declines in physical and cognitive functioning?

OVERVIEW OF THE WORKSHOP

Over the course of the workshop, Lin identified several prominent themes that emerged from the presentations of individual speakers. These themes should not be seen as the conclusions or recommendations of the workshop, but they are presented here to introduce the wide range of topics discussed during the meeting as observed by Lin.

The Links to Healthy Aging

Hearing loss is often treated as an unavoidable and relatively unimportant consequence of aging, yet it clearly contributes to a variety of physical, cognitive, and psychosocial problems. Presently, age-related hearing loss is poorly understood and often stigmatized, not only among patients and consumers but also among the research community and providers, said Lin. Technology and models of care are not meeting the needs of many individuals.

Deficits in Hearing Health Care

According to Lin, hearing health care is fragmented, expensive, and often inadequate. The hearing health care workforce includes not just physicians but also audiologists, hearing aid dispensers, community health workers, and others. Although united by the underlying problem of hearing loss, each group has its own interests and approaches. In addition, third-party reimbursement in the United States for hearing products and services is generally spotty or nonexistent.

The Rapidly Changing State of Hearing Technologies

Although hearing aids, cochlear implants, assistive listening devices, and other technologies have made great advances in recent years, Lin noted, they still fail to meet the needs of many older adults with hearing loss, such as extracting a voice from a noisy environment. At the same time, technology is continuing to advance rapidly, and newer devices, such as hearing loops in public spaces and hearing applications built into smartphones, have tremendous potential to help people hear better.

The Potential for Innovative Approaches

New ways of delivering care and raising awareness of age-related hearing loss could yield major steps forward, stated Lin. Higher levels of screening, enhanced education and counseling, rehabilitation strategies, greater use of community health workers, and outreach campaigns to both the hearing-impaired and general populations could greatly expand the visibility of the issue and the efforts being made to counter hearing loss.

Research Gaps

Lin concluded that much remains unknown about age-related hearing loss, including the relationship between hearing loss and other physical and cognitive deficits, the best ways to deliver hearing health care, and the effects of reimbursement on the use of hearing technologies. Several speakers at the workshop commented on the value that could be derived from a large-scale randomized controlled trial of the association between better hearing health care and healthy aging.

The workshop was designed to catalyze changes that are already ongoing, Lin observed. The aging of the baby boomers, rapid technological advances, changes in the health care system, and recognition of the problems caused by hearing loss are coming together to produce a unique opportunity. As Lin said, the workshop represented "the first time in history that we have had a meeting like this with this many stakeholders at the table." Continued interdisciplinary efforts to address age-related hearing loss could improve the lives of many millions of peoples.

ORGANIZATION OF THE WORKSHOP SUMMARY

This workshop summary is limited to describing the presentations given and general topics discussed during the workshop itself. Overall, each speaker's presentation is captured in a section attributed to that individual. All of the workshop discussions with the audience have also been captured in a variety of ways. For the most part, topics raised and responses given during the discussion periods were incorporated into the individual section for the speaker whose presentation was directly related to the given topic or question. In some cases, where a new topic or line of discussion arose, a separate section was introduced to reflect that new topic. Presentations are also not necessarily organized in the same order as the actual workshop, but have been rearranged to provide a better flow for the readers of this workshop summary.

Following this introductory chapter, Chapter 2 presents the personal experiences of two people with moderate to severe hearing loss who have found ways to overcome these losses and remain healthy and active. Chapter 3 explores the link between hearing and those domains that characterize healthy aging, including physical, cognitive, and psychosocial functioning. Chapter 4 looks at current approaches to hearing health care delivery, both in the United States and abroad. Chapter 5 considers the wealth of rapidly advancing technologies available to counter hearing loss and maintain healthy aging. Chapter 6 describes innovative models to hearing health care, and Chapter 7 looks at some of the most prominent current issues in hearing health care. Finally, Chapter 8 describes collaborative strategies for moving forward, first from the perspectives of several representatives of large organizations and then from the perspectives of individual workshop participants.

2

Hearing Loss: Two Perspectives

During the workshop, two speakers with moderate to severe hearing loss described their experiences and their efforts to remain healthy and socially engaged. Although experiences with hearing loss are as diverse as the people who lose their hearing, these two presentations are summarized here, at the beginning of this report of the workshop, to introduce some of the issues that millions of people deal with every day.

LIVING WITH HEARING LOSS

Katherine Bouton
Author of Shouting Won't Help

Katherine Bouton, a former editor at the *New York Times*, has a hearing aid in her right ear and a cochlear implant on her left ear. "I wear them all day, every day. I wouldn't have a life without them."

Bouton first started losing her hearing when she was 30. Hearing loss is often thought of as a condition of aging, but about two-thirds of people with hearing loss begin to lose their hearing before the age of 60, she observed. If everyone could realize that hearing loss affects people of all ages, Bouton added, we could defeat the stigma of age, and people would be much more likely to wear hearing aids.

Bouton was in denial for many years. She denied that her hearing was bad or that she needed a hearing aid. More than 20 years elapsed after she was given a diagnosis of a fairly severe hearing loss before she obtained hearing aids. Even then, she was sure that her otolaryngologist (also known as an ear, nose, and throat, or ENT, physician) would find the cause of her hearing loss and reverse the progression. But the cause remained undiagnosed, and she began researching hearing loss herself.

Meanwhile, her hearing continued to decline, "and so did my spirits," she said. "I sank deeper and deeper into depression. In 2008, I lost the minimal remaining hearing in my left ear and most of the hearing in my right ear as well. I isolated myself increasingly at work and with friends. I avoided the cafeteria. I avoided meetings I should go to. I never went out for drinks afterwards with people. . . . The night of Obama's first election, I watched the election returns alone at home on my couch," she said, declining an invitation to watch with friends. Bouton admitted she was lonely and drank too much. "I fell asleep before I even knew that Obama had won."

She added, "Always accompanying this depression was anger. There was anger at my hearing, anger at my colleagues, anger at my husband. I was short with my kids. I was estranged from my friends. I was angry with the hearing aid industry for not coming up with better products. I was angry at my audiologist for not being able to make me hear again. I was angry at science. I was angry at the world."

The next year she obtained a cochlear implant, but her experience was not as positive as some. Negative stress and years of neglect made it hard for her to adjust to her implant. Shortly after the implant was activated, she left her job at the *New York Times*. "Despite the cochlear implant and the hearing aid, I really couldn't do [the work I loved]. I wasn't interested in doing the work that was offered as a substitute."

She was unemployed, functionally deaf, and at rock bottom. "Anger actually helped, surprisingly enough. Anger was my original incentive for writing *Shouting Won't Help*. I thought, 'I will show them. I will show them what I have been through. I will show them all how badly they treated me and how unsympathetic they were.' Fortunately, I moved on. That is not a good premise for a book."

As she researched hearing loss and talked with more people with hearing loss, she gradually gained perspective. Eventually, she said, she reached "that elusive stage of acceptance. I was able to accept that hearing loss is part of who I am."

People experience hearing loss in different ways, depending on the degree and the nature of the loss, the kind of correction they have, the kind of person they are, and the relative difficulty of the challenges in their daily hearing environments. For many, whatever the circumstances, hearing loss can be emotionally devastating. "We grieve the loss not only of our hearing but often of our way of life," Bouton said. "Hearing loss affects how we work. It affects our enjoyment of music and movies and lectures, our relationships with family and friends."

Bouton said her hearing loss is like being underwater. It is lonely but peaceful. With her hearing aids and implant, sounds can be very loud, but she can also hear quiet sounds, such as birds chirping and streams gurgling. Most important, she can hear speech. "I can't hear anything without my devices. They are essential to me."

Bouton has come to terms with her hearing loss. "I own my hearing loss. My hearing loss doesn't own me." But she still has fits of what the blogger Gael Hannan calls "ear rage."[1] "Hearing loss is always there and always ready to trip you up," she said.

The Hearing Aid Marketplace

Most consumers find the hearing aid marketplace incredibly frustrating, said Bouton. Many do not know what kind of hearing aid to get, where they should buy it, how well it will work, whether they can afford it, whether they need an audiologist, or how to find a good audiologist. "People are really confused about how even to take the first steps."

Bouton said she has a good audiologist, recommended by her ENT physician, who guided her through the maze. Her first pair of hearing aids cost $6,000 in 2002, which was "a major bite out of my salary." When she applied for insurance reimbursement, she received $500 for the two hearing aids. With three subsequent hearing aids, her insurance did not reimburse her at all. "It is no wonder to me that so many people turn to the big-box stores or the Internet for their hearing aid purchases," she said. "We are a do-it-yourself country when it comes to consumerism. We shop where we can get the best bargain. We have to acknowledge that the Internet and the big-box stores are part of the hearing aid community."

She recommended, however, that even low-cost hearing aids should be accompanied by the services of an audiologist. Her own audiologist spent many hours with her over the years. Her hearing would seem fine in the acoustically ideal environment of her audiologist's office. But when she walked out onto the street, she would be assaulted by street noise, or speech would sound imprecise or fuzzy in the real world. "I would go back. She would fix it."

Even with her audiologist's help, she heard "too much of what I didn't want to hear and not enough of what I did want to hear." Sometimes her hearing aid itched or was too tight or not tight enough. Her audiologist would adjust it or send it back to the manufacturer. Every time she received a new hearing aid, her audiologist immediately scheduled follow-up appointments in the first 30-day period to readjust and reprogram her hearing aid. Still, her experiences with hearing aids were often frustrating. Bouton said that her hearing loss is complicated and that she often had to try differ-

---

[1] See www.gaelhannan.com (accessed May 9, 2014).

ent brands before finding the one that worked best for her. Her audiologist "stuck with me cheerfully through these many, many years of hearing aids," she said. "I am sure that I was far from her most cost-effective patient."

Even exceptional audiologists can have lapses, said Bouton. Her audiologist did not explain that getting the most from a hearing aid takes practice and patience. She did not refer Bouton to a hearing loss support group. She did not tell Bouton about the rehabilitation programs available on the Internet. None of her hearing aids had a telecoil (also known as a T-coil) until 2 years ago when she specifically asked for one. (Telecoils and other technologies are discussed in Chapter 4.) "This isn't unusual—40 percent of hearing aids today still do not have T-coils."

Her audiologist did offer Bouton a variety of assistive listening devices, most of which she turned down as being "too much stuff." Bouton finally bought an iCom Bluetooth for use with her telephone, which worked as long as she was in a quiet place. But the device caused a lag in communications when she used a cell phone. People would say that they could not hear her on the phone, "which I always found ironic since most of the time I can't hear them. Generally, the phone continues to elude me, even with all of the devices I have." She uses captioned phones when she can.

Two years ago, her audiologist provided her with a wireless FM system, which also can be synced to a cell phone. It is much more versatile than the iCom, she said. It can be used in personal conversations by holding it toward someone. It can be put on a podium to hear a lecture. "The first time I used it for any sustained period of time was on a trip I made to China. The guide wore it. It was fabulous. I heard everything he said in crowded marketplaces, in museums." She was "thrilled with it," but she still takes issue with the design. For example, the controls are on the device that goes with the speaker, which "doesn't make any sense. It is me, the listener, who needs to be able to change those controls." The receiver has a small volume control, but there is no way to change the program or the channel. "I am not about to walk up to the podium and start fooling around with it in the middle of somebody's speech." Furthermore, the multiple parts have a tendency to break down, and it is often hard to tell where the flaw is. "Finding out why it doesn't work involves the busy audiologist again and, generally, weeks and weeks of waiting while one part after another is sent back to the manufacturer." At this point, she knows the representatives at the companies that provide many of her technologies, and she works directly with them in finding solutions. Bouton said that the cochlear implant companies use this model, and it eliminates unnecessary steps.

Chargers are another problem. Bouton said she has enough chargers to fill an entire bedside table with equipment. "I do wonder why it is not possible to make something more like a universal charger," she said. "Every charger is different."

In the past few years she has had a chance to experience looping, in which a wire installed around the perimeter of a room sends a signal to the telecoils in hearing aids and cochlear implants. Looping enables her to hear better than any technology she has used before. It does not require extra equipment or another charger. She does not have to put anything around her neck or on her head. She noted that looping does not solve all problems, however. People who are profoundly deaf or do not wear a hearing aid with a telecoil or have an implant cannot benefit from it. Moreover, it cannot be used if people do not know that looping is available. Loop signs should be displayed both inside and outside venues, she said, and venues should advertise on the World Wide Web and in print that they are looped. Furthermore, relatively few venues have installed looping. Consumers do not know what it is and do not ask for it. Even Bouton's audiologist did not know about looping and did not realize how useful it would be for her. "You want more gray hair in your audience? Get that looping system in there."

Future Actions

Bouton also recommended certain actions. She said that standardized best-practice protocols are needed at every level. "The hearing aid marketplace truly is a chaotic mess. Consumers are overwhelmed by the choices and the cost." These types of protocols would benefit the industry by reducing the rate of returns from consumers who have not been educated about their hearing loss, who have not been counseled about the need to come back in for reprogramming, or who have hearing aids that do not fit properly.

Audiologists, social workers, geriatricians, and nursing home employees need to understand the emotional toll that hearing loss takes, she said. They would then be better able to empathize with those who express anger and could encourage people to join support groups. They could even turn a negative into a positive by encouraging these individuals to become advocates for people with hearing loss.

Every audiologist should offer the same minimum checklist of services, said Bouton; for example, ideally, hearing aids need to be tested in a real-world environment. Bouton urged hearing aid companies to develop products that work even in noise, make assistive devices that are simple to use, and bring their prices in line with other consumer electronics. "I think we are all baffled by why this is not possible."

The government needs to mandate coverage for hearing aids, said Bouton. The cost of not providing hearing aids is far higher in terms of unemployment and in cognitive decline than the cost of providing them.

"Hearing aids should be as common, as effective, as affordable, and as unremarkable as glasses," Bouton concluded.

HEARING TECHNOLOGIES FROM A CONSUMER PERSPECTIVE

Richard Einhorn
Composer of Voices of Light

Richard Einhorn is a recording engineer, a Grammy-winning former record producer, and a composer. His composition *Voices of Light* has been performed all over the world and was scheduled to be performed at the Kennedy Center in Washington, DC, a few weeks after the workshop. In the middle of his career, Einhorn experienced a sudden and severe hearing loss. "Sound has always been the primary way I orient myself to the world," he said. "Now that I live with a very serious hearing loss, my quest to hear better has taken on a special urgency. Hearing better is absolutely essential for my mental and physical well-being. That is something I don't know from studies, but I know simply as part of who I am."

Einhorn said that he is essentially deaf in his right ear and has a 60 dB conductive loss from otosclerosis in his left ear. "It is a terrible thing to live with this condition, and it has affected every single part of my life, except, interestingly enough, composing, which is primarily an act of the imagination." At the workshop, he played an example of what his hearing sounds like, and he said that the sound is so unbearable that he normally wears an earplug in his right ear.[2]

Einhorn described the technologies he uses to overcome his hearing loss, focusing both on how well the technologies work and on how easy and comfortable they are to use. He did not discuss looping technologies at the workshop, though he has been a prominent advocate for their installation.

The technology and ergonomics of hearing aids and personal sound amplifier products have become extremely good, he said, but "the truth is that many users, including myself, are less than satisfied with the performance of hearing aids in noisy situations." The basic problem is the inadequate acoustic technique used in hearing aids. When the microphone is placed on or in the ears, it is too far away from the desired sound source to pick up a clean enough signal to extract speech from noise. Furthermore, the processing power inside a hearing aid is too limited to extract the signal.

The solution is to get the microphone closer to the signal, which can be done through assistive listening devices (ALDs). Common types include

---

[2] The archived video webcast of Einhorn's presentation, including the example he played, is available at http://www.iom.edu/Activities/PublicHealth/HearingLossAging/2014-JAN-13. aspx (accessed February 25, 2014).

portable microphones connected to amplifiers and wireless transmitters that can send the signal from a microphone to a receiver. "The idea then is that somebody can be holding this [microphone] and talking to you, or you can put it on a lectern." ALDs also can send a signal to a telecoil in a hearing aid through a wire loop worn around the neck.

A common problem with these systems, said Einhorn, is that they are not robust enough. Telecoils tend to hum in electrically ungrounded settings or other environments that are not well engineered. "If you don't know that your environment is hum-free, you cannot reliably depend upon using a neck loop." To overcome this problem, hearing aid companies have created integrated systems that use different technologies to send signals to hearing aids. They tend to be expensive and proprietary, however, which makes it difficult or impossible to replace parts of the system, such as a microphone, with a preferred technology. Another problem with ALDs is that they require carrying around "a whole bunch of stuff," said Einhorn. "They are essentially a Rube Goldberg contraption."

A technology that could solve many of these problems, he continued, is the smartphone. They are very powerful computers with a microphone, an amplifier, and a sound output. "In fact, for some of them—for example, the iPhone—the sound quality is just below professional quality." People already have them in their pockets, which means they do not have to carry around a lot of additional equipment. And they can be modified to assist with hearing loss. Einhorn has developed a system in which he has replaced the standard earbuds with a set of very good earphones and has installed a hearing aid application on his phone, resulting in a very high-quality hearing assistance device.

"It is like Galileo with the telescope," he said. "People who have tried it, including people with severe hearing loss, have told me that this system works. There is starting to be peer review of this technology, and it basically bears out what I am telling you anecdotally."

Further refinements could include directional microphones, wireless transmission to hearing aids, and further signal processing. "Is this a pipe dream? Well, I thought it was 3 years ago, when I first realized that it could be done," he said. But tremendous progress has occurred since then, to the point that smartphones now could become the hub of a transparent assistive listening system.

"Hearing loss, of course, is a medical problem," Einhorn concluded. "Hearing better—as well as your ears will allow—is essentially an acoustical and ergonomics problem. Present hearing technology is often not adequate because it doesn't address the acoustic and ergonomics problems in a holistic way. A new approach to hearing assistance, based on smartphones, could dramatically improve the ability of millions of people to hear."

3

The Connection Between Hearing Loss and Healthy Aging

The physical, cognitive, psychological, and psychosocial consequences of hearing loss were a prominent topic at the workshop. This chapter brings together six presentations that focused on these issues. Together, they demonstrate that hearing loss is not only a pervasive problem but also one that can affect virtually all aspects of a person's life.

THE CONSEQUENCES OF UNTREATED HEARING LOSS

James Firman
National Council on Aging

Jim Firman has had a hearing loss his whole life.[1] "I understand, at a personal level, the benefits and limitations of treatment," he said. In addition, as president and chief executive officer of the National Council on Aging, an organization whose mission is to improve the lives of millions of older adults, he is alarmed by both the prevalence and the consequences of untreated hearing loss.

First, he observed, hearing loss is very common. Firman said that 2 of every 100 children have hearing loss, as does 1 of 14 people under age 65. Of people between the ages of 65 and 84, he said 40 percent have hearing losses, as do 2 of 3 people over the age of 85.

---

[1] Firman demonstrates what his hearing sounds like in the video of his presentation, which is available at http://www.iom.edu/Activities/PublicHealth/HearingLossAging/2014-JAN-13. aspx (accessed February 24, 2014).

Hearing loss is also invisible. No one can tell that people have a hearing loss or the severity of the loss by looking at them. "You have really no idea what it means to them," Firman said. In addition, hearing loss is invisible to many who have hearing loss. They are aware that they are missing things, but they do not have a clear idea of how much or what they have missed. They do not know how much they do not hear of what their bosses, their coworkers, their spouses, their children, or their grandchildren are saying. "Most people with hearing loss do not understand what they are missing, and, therefore, they are not motivated to take action."

Hearing loss is also insidious. The consequences are not obvious, but they can have psychophysical, cognitive, and psychosocial impacts. Most important, said Firman, the inability to communicate well makes it much harder to remain an active, engaged, and contributing member of society. For example, he recounted an episode where he was unable to hear his adult son ask whether he wanted to go out for dinner. "It is the insidious, subtle consequences in everyday situations where we need to focus the most attention."

Finally, hearing loss is treatable, he said. Even people with severe hearing loss can function at a much higher level with proper hearing aids and treatment. Firman himself relies not only on good hearing aids but also on good speech-reading skills. If he closes his eyes, he can miss half of what a person is saying. "If we want to correct this problem among older adults, it is not just about amplification. It is about auditory training and speech reading as well."

Barriers to Treatment

Yet hearing loss often remains untreated. Nine of ten people with mild loss do not have hearing aids, Firman observed. Six of 10 people with moderate to severe hearing loss do not have hearing aids, and 70 percent of people between age 65 and 84 do not use hearing aids. Firman described a study conducted by the National Council on Aging in 1999 on the consequences of hearing loss in older adults—he noted that 69 percent of the people with untreated hearing loss said that their hearing was not bad enough to require a hearing aid. "I can guarantee you, as a person with a moderate to severe loss, that there is no way that you are doing fine and getting along fine if that hearing loss is not treated."

One of five people in the survey also said that wearing a hearing aid would make them feel old or embarrassed. Yet they are not too embarrassed to respond inappropriately, to withdraw from situations, or to be viewed as senile, said Firman. "This is just astounding to me."

Hearing loss is not a priority for policy makers, Firman observed. They are not seriously talking about expanding coverage for hearing aids. Policy makers and the general public are unsure about whether hearing loss is a lifestyle issue, a health care cost issue, or a public health concern. Medicaid, which has provided some coverage for hearing aids in the past, may be cutting back because of cost pressures, despite the cost-effectiveness of hearing aids. Only the U.S. Department of Veterans Affairs has steadfastly supported their use.

Finally, hearing loss is a solvable public health challenge, he said. Interventions exist and work. "What we have to do is create the awareness of the problem and move together with collective action to make a difference." This workshop, Firman concluded, could mark a historic turning point for age-related hearing loss.

THE IMPACT OF HEARING LOSS ON PHYSICAL FUNCTIONING

Alan M. Jette
Boston University School of Public Health

Hearing loss is seen by many people to be a communication disorder, but it may have much more wide-ranging consequences. It could increase the risk of falls and injuries, lead to increased functional limitation and subsequent disability, and reduce one's activity and participation, leading to decreased quality of life.

Alan Jette, director of Boston University's Health and Disability Research Institute, reviewed some recent longitudinal studies on the potential functional consequences of hearing loss. With regard to falls, a study of twins in Finland hypothesized that postural balance would act as an important mediator between hearing loss and falls. In a study of 423 women with a mean age of 68 years, rates of falls for the best to the poorest hearing quartiles were 7.1, 6.7, 10.4, and 11.3 falls per 100 person-months (Viljanen et al., 2009). In the poorest hearing group, 30 percent reported two or more falls versus 17 percent in the best hearing group. Even after controlling for postural balance, those with poor hearing still had a twofold increased risk of falls. The same study looked at the impact of hearing loss on walking ability. Of 434 women ages 63 to 76, 41 percent of those with impaired hearing correlated cross-sectionally with poor mobility. In age-adjusted logistic regression, the women with hearing loss had twice the risk for new major difficulties in walking 2 kilometers as those without hearing loss.

The Health ABC study, which is a population-based study of 3,000 individuals ages 70 years and older, has also looked at the association of age-related hearing loss with function and disability. In a prospective cohort study of more than 2,200 adults ages 70 to 79 (Chen et al., in review), observed a small "dose-dependent" effect of hearing with functional loss, with greater levels of hearing loss associated with poorer function over time and, among women, greater risk for incident disability. Results were robust to adjustment for multiple potential confounders. Women with moderate or greater hearing loss had a 31 percent greater increased risk of disability compared with those with normal hearing. This association was not seen for men in this cohort study.

Fully adjusted analyses restricted to individuals with mild or greater hearing loss found that individuals who used hearing aids had functional scores that were not significantly different from individuals not using hearing aids. Hearing aid use also brought no significant attenuation in the risk of incident disability. Nevertheless, data on key variables—such as the hours a hearing aid was worn per day, the number of years used, and the adequacy of rehabilitation—that may affect the success of hearing rehabilitation and any observed association were not available in the Health ABC study.

Another study in Alameda County, California looked at the association of hearing loss with the ability to perform activities of daily living (ADLs), instrumental activities of daily living (IADLs), physical performance, depression, and social participation. A 1-year prospective cohort study in a sample of about 2,500 people found no consistent association between hearing loss and performance of ADLs, IADLs, or physical performance (Wallhagen et al., 2001). The study did, however, see a clear association with social functioning, as measured by feeling left out, feeling lonely or remote, finding difficulty in feeling close to others, or not being able to pay attention, with the association higher for those with moderate and severe hearing loss as opposed to mild hearing loss.

Finally, Jette discussed the association between hearing loss and driving behaviors. Research has shown that people with hearing impairments are more likely to have ceased driving (Gilhotra et al., 2001). In a study from Quebec that used a database of driving records, daily noise exposure and measured hearing loss were associated with greater risk of traffic accidents (Picard et al., 2008). And a study from Australia found that people with moderate to severe hearing impairment had significantly poorer driving performance in the presence of auditory distractors (being asked to report sums of numbers) as compared to those with normal or mild hearing impairment (Hickson et al., 2010).

In summary, existing studies on the association of hearing loss with functional decline are inconsistent, Jette said. Some demonstrate a positive association. Others find weak or no significant association. The results depend on such factors as which function is being examined and how hearing loss is measured. Nevertheless, Jette said, on the basis of available literature, hearing loss appears to have some real but relatively modest functional and disability consequences that could affect one's quality of life. Still, he noted, "the state of the science is far from mature." For example, the literature has not examined associated factors, such as who can afford an expensive hearing aid and the degree to which hearing aids are worn.

In the future, the exposure variable of greatest interest needs to be clarified, Jette observed. Uncorrected hearing loss is most commonly assessed, which seems appropriate when the focus is on the impact of hearing loss on outcomes such as falls and functional limitations. When the focus is on disability behaviors such as driving and social participation, however, hearing loss with correction may be the more meaningful exposure variable. As other speakers noted, a critical and fascinating question is whether hearing aid use or other forms of correction have a modifying effect on associations with physical functioning. Careful observational studies with and without correction could pave the way for controlled trials. Also, although the functional measures may seem simple, in fact functional outcomes are complex, and work is needed to clarify those most related to hearing loss, Jette said. One's capacity to perform key functional tasks such as walking and to prevent events such as falls is critical to explore as well.

FUNCTIONAL RESERVES AND HEARING

Luigi Ferrucci
National Institute on Aging

As people age, their bodies continually adjust and compensate to maintain good physical and cognitive function, observed Luigi Ferrucci, scientific director of the National Institute on Aging. But when physical and cognitive reserves are depleted and compensation no longer works, declines can follow. Some individuals maintain a high level of functioning up to the last day of their lives. Others start showing functional decline much earlier because of disease or other causes. Extending good function to these latter individuals represents a tremendous public health opportunity.

In addition, hearing loss can have enormous personal consequences. Ferrucci recounted a conversation with a group of centenarians, most of whom had hearing loss, who reported that hearing loss was their number one concern. They were afraid that something was going to happen and that they would not be able to react because they could not hear.

Ferrucci and Studenski (2011) have defined four aging phenotypes that contribute to the genesis of geriatric syndromes:

- Changes in body composition
- Energy imbalance in production or utilization
- Homeostatic dysregulation
- Neurodegeneration

In his presentation, Ferrucci focused on energy imbalances, though he said that hearing loss can have effects across all four domains. A healthy person expends 60 to 70 percent of the energy used each day simply carrying out the body's basic functions, he said. Someone fighting disease or disability uses even more energy to maintain this homeostatic equilibrium. Instability, infirmity, or inefficiency can further eat into energy stores. As a result, such individuals have less energy for other activities, such as movement or thinking.

The brain has a variety of activities to which it must devote resources, including attention, cognitive function, motor function, balance, hearing, vision, cardiovascular control, and metabolic control. Dual tasks create a competition for brain resources. For example, people talking on their cell phones tend to walk more slowly, and organists know that using the organ's pedals makes it very difficult to play the keyboard quickly. In young and healthy individuals, additional resources can be pulled from reserves. But in older individuals, functional resources are constrained, which can lead to dysfunction.

When people have trouble hearing, they have to spend more energy to understand what is coming from their ears. Older people also have less functional reserve that they can allocate to this task. As a result, they can have trouble dealing with a separate but simultaneous task, such as walking or dealing with a sudden obstacle. "The entire range of your functional status is going to be affected," said Ferrucci.

From these observations, Ferrucci drew four conclusions:

- Older age is often associated with a state of brain susceptibility, reduced plasticity, and diminished functional reserve.
- Additional requests to the brain compete with finite resources, which may have functional consequences and increase fragility.
- Because of reduced plasticity, effective adaptation is less likely to occur.
- Hearing loss may have a negative impact on unexpected functional domains.

AGING AND HEARING LOSS: WHY DOES IT MATTER?

Kathleen Pichora-Fuller
University of Toronto

When you are hard of hearing you struggle to hear;
When you struggle to hear you get tired;
When you get tired you get frustrated;
When you get frustrated you get bored;
When you get bored you quit.
—I didn't quit today.

Not everyone is as successful as this acquaintance of Kathleen Pichora-Fuller, professor of psychology at the University of Toronto. Many people respond to this cascade from hearing issues to cognitive issues to emotional issues to social issues by simply withdrawing from social interaction. She noted that this is "absolutely not" what we want to happen to people.

People have many different kinds of hearing loss, Pichora-Fuller said. People can have an audiogram that would not suggest hearing problems, yet they can still have hearing deficits. They may be able to hear someone in ideal listening conditions, where it is quiet, they are listening to just one speaker, the person and topic are familiar, and they are able to focus their attention on the conversation. But in challenging listening conditions—where it is noisy, many people are talking, people have accents or speak quickly, the topic is unfamiliar, or a listener is multitasking or getting used to a new hearing aid—they can have much more difficulty. This can especially be a problem in health care or emergency situations where people need to understand what they are being told.

Older people can particularly have trouble with speech perception in noise, Pichora-Fuller noted. In one test, listeners heard 50 sentences with varying levels of noise and were asked to repeat each sentence's final word (Pichora-Fuller et al., 1995). Half the sentences had contextual clues about what the final word would be: "Stir your coffee with a spoon." The other sentences did not provide a helpful context: "John did not talk about the spoon." Older people with good audiograms needed about 3 dB better signal-to-noise ratio to understand the same number of words. Nonetheless, the older people derived more benefit from the context—again, about a 3 dB difference in the signal-to-noise ratio. Thus, the younger and the older listeners were arriving at about the same performance level but were doing it in different ways. Younger people were more proficient at using the signal, and older people were more proficient at using context.

Age contributes to changes in both hearing and memory, Pichora-Fuller pointed out. In addition, people with lower performance on both memory and hearing measurements tend to attach greater stigma to aging, and hearing problems can result in reduced social participation. The current challenge, she said, is to unpack the connections among these domains using various research approaches and to use new knowledge to inform practice.

Pichora-Fuller stated that hearing loss can have serious widespread health implications in terms of promoting healthy aging. "How do we save people from adverse events that they are likely to encounter because of communication problems?" she asked. "How do we facilitate their ability to self-manage health issues? How do we get them to adhere to and benefit from interventions for health issues that rely on communication?"

Many solutions already exist, and others will be developed through continued research and development. But the solutions need to be combined in a broader perspective that includes the sensory, cognitive, social, and environmental domains, Pichora-Fuller said. For example, hospitals and other health care environments can be extremely noisy. Standards for communication accessibility in such facilities could greatly benefit those with hearing problems.

THE IMPACT OF HEARING LOSS ON COGNITION

Marilyn Albert
Johns Hopkins University School of Medicine

Studies are limited but suggestive of the connection between hearing loss and cognition, noted Marilyn Albert, professor of neurology at the Johns Hopkins University School of Medicine. Two longitudinal studies have demonstrated an association between hearing loss and cognitive decline (Lin et al., 2013; Uhlmann et al., 1989), and two others have demonstrated an association with dementia (Gallacher et al., 2012; Lin et al., 2011b). One is part of the Health ABC study. Using a digit-symbol substitution test to measure cognition, in which people write a symbol for each digit on a piece of paper to measure psychomotor speed, executive function, incidental memory, and attention, individuals who had normal hearing performed much better than individuals who had hearing loss (Lin et al., 2013). The data are "striking," said Albert. "Individuals, even adjusted for level of hearing loss over time, are performing more poorly on this test that doesn't require that you actually hear."

The other longitudinal study Albert described is from the Baltimore Longitudinal Study on Aging, a prospective study of older adults that began in 1958. In 639 individuals followed for more than 10 years, those with hearing loss had a higher probability of developing dementia, with the probability rising with the severity of hearing loss (Lin et al., 2011b). In this study, dementia was defined as progressive declines in mental ability to the point of not being able to function independently, with impairments in two or more domains of cognition. The relationship between hearing loss and time to develop dementia is "convincing and striking," said Albert.

Imaging studies of brain structure have also demonstrated an association with hearing loss. For example, Peelle et al. (2011) showed that poorer hearing is associated with reduced gray matter in the auditory cortices. In addition, Lin et al. (in press), in research on 126 individuals involved in the Baltimore Longitudinal Study on Aging, found a greater loss of mean gray matter volume over time in those with hearing loss versus those who did not lose hearing. Most important, said Albert, the losses occur not just in the brain regions related to hearing but more globally, suggesting that "there is a cascading effect."

Albert hypothesized that two mechanisms could be at work to explain these associations. First, hearing loss could be causing increased brain atrophy. Second, in people with progressive accumulations of brain pathology due to other causes, such as Alzheimer's disease or microvascular disease, two pathological processes could be superimposed. These two pathological processes could contribute to declines in cognition and result in crossing a threshold for dementia at an earlier time.

The loss of hearing is obviously modifiable, Albert said. Therefore, a randomized controlled trial in which some individuals were given hearing aids and followed over time along with individuals who did not have hearing aids could demonstrate the effects of hearing loss on cognition and brain volumes, as well as on such factors as social engagement and quality of life, she concluded.

PSYCHOSOCIAL IMPACTS

Barbara E. Weinstein
Graduate School and University Center, City University of New York

Much more information has recently become available on the psychosocial impacts of hearing loss. Barbara E. Weinstein, professor of audiology and speech language hearing sciences at the City University of New York, provided a brief review of the literature.

Many studies' samples are available from countries around the world, including the following:

- Blue Mountains Hearing Study: a population-based survey of age-related hearing loss in a representative older Australian community;
- Blue Mountains Eye Study: a population-based study of vision and eye diseases among a representative sample of the older Australian community;
- Survey of Disability, Aging and Careers: a national household survey of 43,233 respondents with and without disability using the Australian Bureau of Statistics;
- Program of Education and Aid for the Community-Dwelling Elderly: a field study of health parameters of community-based older people in Japan;
- National Health and Nutrition Examination Study: a program of studies designed to assess the health and nutritional status of adults and children in the United States;
- Epidemiology of Hearing Loss Study: a population-based longitudinal study of age-related hearing loss of people living in Wisconsin; and

- Medicare Current Beneficiary Statement: a continuous multipur-
  pose survey of a nationally representative sample of older persons
  with disabilities, and institutionalized beneficiaries.

The functional disabilities reviewed by Jette have major psychosocial impacts, Weinstein noted. For example, Genther et al. (2013) found that people with mild to profound hearing impairments were more likely to have a history of hospitalizations and hospitalization in the past year. Hearing loss was significantly and independently associated with increased health care use, including the number of hospitalizations. And hearing loss was significantly associated with self-reported poor physical and mental health.

Research has also demonstrated a link between hearing loss and social isolation. Weinstein and Ventry (1982) found that people who were socially isolated had a greater self-perceived hearing disability, worse auditory processing difficulties, and poorer hearing. The correlation was stronger with subjective than objective measures of social isolation, and the strongest relationship was with the self-reported hearing disability. In doing this research, Weinstein said that she broke her sample into groups, and the people who were most subjectively and most objectively isolated were the ones with the worst-measured hearing, the greatest self-perceived hearing disability, and the most challenges in auditory processing.

In a more recent study, Hawthorne (2008) found that the likelihood of self-perceived social isolation increased with the number of chronic conditions. Of note, depression had the strongest association with subjective social isolation, followed by self-reported hearing difficulties. Hearing difficulties came up before vision as a correlate of social isolation.

Depression is prevalent in the elderly, with 15 to 20 percent of older adults having been diagnosed with the condition. Like hearing loss, depression is often undetected and untreated. In a study from Canada, MacDonald (2011) found a strong relationship between self-reported hearing problems and depression. Saito et al. (2010), in a study conducted in Japan, found that the odds of depressive symptoms were high in people with self-reported hearing disability as compared to those without hearing disability. Gopinath et al. (2012) also found an independent association between hearing disability and the presence of depressive symptoms after adjusting for age, sex, walking disability, receipt of pension payment, use of community support services, living alone, cognitive impairment, and history of arthritis or stroke.

Hearing loss affects independence by increasing the reliance on support systems, Weinstein stated. Schneider et al. (2010) demonstrated that hearing loss was associated with increased use of community and informal support systems and was a predictor of use of community support after 5 years. In addition, the severity of hearing loss mattered, with people having moderate to severe hearing loss at increased risk for the need to use community support services. People who used support systems were more likely to be hearing aid users, however.

Hearing loss may also be a risk factor for mortality. Karpa et al. (2010) found that hearing loss severity was connected to mortality, but this connection occurred through mediating variables, including walking difficulty and cognitive impairment. This indirect correlation needs to be considered when thinking about the effectiveness of interventions, Weinstein said.

Finally, hearing loss affects quality of life, including a person's perceptions of health, social interactions, physical function, and psychological function. For example, Dalton et al. (2003) found that self-reported hearing disability and severity of hearing loss was associated with reduced scores on several domains of the SF-36, which is a widely used survey of functional health and well-being. Chia et al. (2007) produced similar results and also showed that the severity and type of hearing loss affect self-reported measures of well-being. Gopinath et al. (2012) also showed that people who developed incident hearing loss were much more likely to have a reduced quality of life.

Weinstein ended on a more positive note. People are more likely to use a hearing aid if they perceive a need for improved hearing, feel disabled by hearing loss, or feel that hearing loss limits their participation in society. Hearing aid users are more likely to score slightly better on the physical summary scores of the SF-36 (Chia et al., 2007), to use and need support services (Schneider et al., 2010), to show significant improvement on the mental domain items of the SF-36 (Gopinath et al., 2012), and to exhibit less decline in the vitality domain than people who do not use hearing aids (Gopinath et al., 2012). Hogan et al. (2009) also found that hearing aid users had a better average quality of life than non-hearing-aid users, though they had a poorer average quality of life than the general population.

Weinstein posed two questions at the end of her talk. What are the absolute and relative risk reductions of hearing interventions, and what is the length of time needed to accrue a clinically meaningful risk reduction in health outcomes associated with hearing difficulties?

Among the most important goals of healthy aging are independence, psychological well-being, successful life course transitions, and self-reported health, Weinstein said. Hearing affects all these measures. "The ability to hear and understand really matters," she concluded.

OTHER ISSUES

During the question-and-answer period, several issues arose which were distinct from the presentations above and so are reflected here.

Research Issues

Weinstein and Albert agreed that there is a great need for randomized controlled trials on the efficacy of hearing aids in improving health outcomes, especially because so much of the data available today remain correlational rather than causative. Weinstein added that the U.S. Preventive Services Task Force did not endorse screening for hearing loss or for cognitive decline, partly because studies have not been conducted demonstrating that interventions will have a beneficial effect relative to screening outcomes. It is also important, Weinstein added, that the efficacy of hearing aids in improving hearing quality of care and life be measured, because people with hearing aids have other health-related issues as well.

Margaret Wallhagen, University of California, San Francisco, who spoke later in the workshop, raised a concern about the ethics of randomized controlled trials if someone is not provided with a useful intervention. Observational studies are able to produce solid findings, as with cigarette smoking and cancer. Causative information is important, and randomized controlled trials are usually the gold standard, but creative research designs also can yield useful information.

Ferrucci emphasized the importance of being able to tell who will do well and who will not do well with a hearing aid. Also, the correlation of hearing loss with medical conditions provides an opening to involve primary care physicians in hearing issues. Jette added that community participation is another important factor. Important social roles can be severely compromised by hearing loss, and these societal roles deserve much more investigation.

Firman pointed out that trials should look not just at the efficacy of hearing aids but also at other forms of hearing rehabilitation, such as speech reading.

Diversity and Accessibility Issues

On a more provocative note, Firman said that much of the research on hearing and healthy aging can be seen as ageist. It starts with the assumption that the most important issue is enabling people to maintain physical or psychosocial function, but the more important questions involve their ability to work. "We know that one-third of older people have to work. They don't have financial resources to do otherwise." Similarly, to what extent are older people able to volunteer or participate in informal family care? he asked. "If we start with the view that this is just about nonfunctioning people who are not expected to contribute to society, that is an ageist point of view. We have to turn this around and say, 'We have this tremendous resource of 78 million people as the baby boomers are growing older. The most important imperative is to keep them working and contributing.'"

Pichora-Fuller observed that hearing problems are very diverse, which means that no one solution is sufficient. This diversity creates problems for clinicians, who have to decide how best to help their patients. For example, perhaps the many people with hearing loss who do not use hearing aids need different kinds of solutions. Diversity also complicates the question of when interventions should be undertaken. In an analogy with hypertension, clinicians do not want to wait for someone to have a heart attack before they start educating that person about changing lifestyles and taking other soft interventions. This question, said Albert, is the kind of problem that randomized controlled trials can address.

Pichora-Fuller also recounted some advice she once received from someone in a wheelchair. He recommended not talking about *hearing loss* because that made the problem too narrow of an issue to appeal to the population as a whole. A far better approach, he said, is to talk about *communication accessibility* in the spirit of universal design (see Chapter 6) to ensure that everyone has an environment that is conducive to communicating.

4

Current Approaches to Hearing
Health Care Delivery

The system for delivering hearing health care is undergoing dramatic changes. Traditionally, patients would be referred from a primary care physician to an ENT physician or an audiologist, who would examine patients and provide them with a hearing aid or other device. Today, the traditional system is being supplemented by sales over the Internet and through big-box stores, telemedicine, and direct-to-consumer advertising.

Three speakers at the workshop examined the hearing health care system in the United States and abroad. Innovations in the system are covered both in this chapter and in Chapter 6.

THE SPECTRUM OF HEARING IMPAIRMENT
AND INTERVENTIONS

Theresa Hnath Chisolm
University of South Florida

Age-related hearing loss, also known as presbycusis, can have many different impacts on a person, explained Theresa Hnath Chisolm, professor and chair of the Department of Communication Sciences and Disorders at the University of South Florida. It is associated with elevated hearing thresholds, so people cannot hear soft sounds. It reduces speech understanding in noisy and echoing environments. And it can interfere with the perception of rapid changes in speech, leading to such complaints as "I can hear people talking but can't understand what they are saying," or "If they spoke slower (or clearer), I could understand what they are saying."

As previous speakers noted (see Chapter 3), age-related hearing loss is associated with sadness and depression, worry, anxiety, emotional turmoil, and insecurity, said Chisolm. What is interesting, too, she added, the symptoms of untreated hearing loss are remarkably similar to those of Alzheimer's disease. As has been attributed to Helen Keller, "Blindness separates us from things, but deafness separates us from people."[1] Nevertheless, hearing loss can be effectively managed so that people can continue to live full and active lives. Managing for healthy hearing begins with identification, Chisolm observed. But it also is associated with having individuals believe that hearing is important and that hearing loss can be treated effectively.

The American Academy of Audiology has produced a document titled *Guidelines for the Audiological Management of Adult Hearing Impairment* (Valente et al., 2006), and these guidelines have been supplemented by subsequent research. These evidence-based protocols begin with a comprehensive assessment of the hearing impairment, functional hearing-related difficulties, and individual factors shown by research to affect intervention. Once any medically treatable hearing losses are ruled out, an integrated treatment plan is developed that has both technical and nontechnical aspects. The outcomes of the interventions are then measured, and the resulting information is used to modify the treatment plan.

Assessing Hearing Loss

As Chisolm explained, an audiogram shows how sensitive an individual's hearing is to different sounds that range from low pitch to high pitch, with the degree of hearing loss ranging from mild to profound. Still, the pure-tone average, which is calculated by averaging sensitivity thresholds for specific frequencies, is only one component of hearing loss. Another component is distortion, which results in problems with the clarity or the cleanness of the signals. Making sounds louder does not necessarily increase their clarity. In addition, external factors such as noise and reverberation or echoing can obscure speech sounds and affect how well hearing aids and other devices work in a given environment. Reverberation off walls and other surfaces, for instance, can create a great deal of difficulty for listeners. And for every doubling of distance, a sound signal loses 6 dB in intensity. All these difficulties are exacerbated by the effects of hearing loss in aging and by age-related cognitive processing declines.

Managing hearing loss requires not just an audiogram but a measure

---

[1] See http://libguides.gallaudet.edu/content.php?pid=352126&sid=2881882 (accessed March 14, 2014).

of a person's ability to understand speech in noise, Chisolm continued. Many objective measures of speech-in-noise are available, but they are not always used in the clinic. These measures yield a signal-to-noise ratio that an individual needs to understand about 50 percent of the speech. A person with normal hearing typically needs the speech to be 2 dB louder than the noise for 50 percent correct recognition. A person with hearing loss might need speech to be 12 dB or more above the noise for 50 percent correct recognition. Unfortunately, this measure cannot be predicted just from an audiogram.

In addition to an audiogram and a signal-to-noise ratio for 50 percent correct recognition, functional hearing-related difficulties need to be assessed. This assessment can be done through a detailed case history, but that case history should not necessarily focus on the medical aspects related to the person's hearing loss, Chisolm said. Rather, the case history should center on what it is like for that person to live with the hearing loss daily and the social and emotional impact of that hearing loss. Many psychometrically valid self-report measures can provide useful information for documenting and identifying the restrictions in activity limitations and participation restrictions that are associated with hearing loss; one of the most widely used measures is the Hearing Handicap Inventory for the Elderly (Ventry and Weinstein, 1982). Other individual factors also need to be examined. For example, research shows that cognition, expectations, motivation, willingness to take risks, assertiveness, manual dexterity, visual acuity, general health, tinnitus, occupational demands, and the presence of support systems can impinge on decisions for intervention and the outcomes of intervention.

Once the results of a comprehensive assessment are available, appropriate treatment goals for a person can be developed. These treatment goals must be individualized, said Chisolm. "One size does not fit all for a person with hearing loss." Chisolm uses the Client Oriented Scale of Improvement (Dillon et al., 1997). This tool, which was developed at the National Acoustic Laboratories in Australia, calls for establishing three to five realistic and achievable intervention goals. Progress toward these goals then can be measured after the intervention has been initiated and used to modify the plan.

Kinds of Interventions

Interventions can be technical or nontechnical. In the former category, most people with mild to moderate hearing losses can be effectively helped through the use of hearing aids. Fitting a hearing aid is not a simple process, Chisolm reminded the workshop participants. Many evidence-based decisions involving features, style, signal processing, and so on need to be made. Then, once an individual is fitted with a hearing aid, the fit needs to be checked in terms of both the amplification characteristics and the physical fit and comfort to the individual.

As described in the previous chapter, hearing aid interventions can improve emotional, social, cognitive, and communication functioning (Mulrow et al., 1990). Davis et al. (2007) also demonstrated a higher quality of life as a function of hearing level in new referrals before and after being fitted with a hearing aid.

Hearing aids provide limited help for most people with more severe to profound hearing impairments. Cochlear implants, however, which bypass the defective cochlea of the ear and directly stimulate the acoustic nerve, provide a very efficacious intervention, said Chisolm. These devices are surgically implanted electrode arrays with external signal processors, and they have been shown to improve speech perception and quality of life (Klop et al., 2007). Still, even with the best hearing aids or cochlear implants, the combined effects of noise, reverberation, and distance continue to represent challenges for listening and communicating for many individuals with hearing loss.

Intervention with assistive listening technologies, such as the loops used in public spaces (these technologies are discussed in more detail in Chapter 5), are important in meeting the challenges of listening in poor listening environments. These technologies can be used alone or combined with hearing aids and cochlear implants to supplement performance in a variety of difficult listening conditions. With these devices, sound is picked up and transmitted directly to the listener, thus overcoming deterioration resulting from noise, reverberation, and distance. They catch the sounds that are important to a person, carry the sounds through a hard wire or wireless link to the listener, and couple the sounds to the listener's ear. A variety of alerting devices that convey either a visual or tactile signal are also available. But effective use of any technology requires systematic device orientation and instruction regarding use and care, either individually or in groups. And usually this instruction needs to occur more than once, because only about 50 percent of medical information is typically remembered by individuals, said Chisolm.

Nontechnical intervention is often called aural or audiological rehabilitation. Typically, in group-based aural rehabilitation programs, participants learn about communication strategies, problem-solving approaches, assistive listening devices, information and advice to give their significant communication partners, and relaxation techniques. Ideally, after getting to know about these techniques, people can try out the various approaches and report back to the clinician about what was successful and what was difficult. Chisolm and Arnold (2012) recently reviewed the evidence for the effectiveness of group-based aural rehabilitation and found good evidence that some of these approaches could improve outcomes for individuals with hearing loss. In particular, the group produced reduced perceptions of disability and improvements on many quality-of-life measures. Group aural rehabilitation programs can bring benefits much quicker than if an individual were given a hearing aid without the provision of such follow-up care. In addition, communications partners benefit if they participate in the programs; for example, they can come to understand why they should not talk to a spouse sitting in the living room watching television while they are in the kitchen washing the dishes. Providing information and counseling about communication strategies can be helpful even for those with mild hearing losses who might not be ready to use hearing aids or other forms of personal amplification.

Another type of aural rehabilitation involves listening or auditory training. Many commercially available computer-based auditory training systems are available. Nonetheless, even though some evidence suggests that these approaches might be helpful, the latest systematic review of computer-based auditory training systems for adults with hearing loss found that the efficacy of these programs is not robust enough to recommend this approach for all patients (Henshaw and Ferguson, 2013). Further research is needed for optimizing auditory training for adults with hearing loss, Chisolm observed.

A Public Health Perspective

From a public health perspective, the optimum situation would be for individuals to recognize that they have impaired hearing, for society and individuals to believe it is important and should be treated, and for effective treatments to be readily accessible, Chisolm said. Today, however, age-related hearing loss is not understood to be an important public health issue. Studies of cognitive, functional, and social-emotional effects need to continue, she said, along with studies examining health beliefs and attitudes about hearing loss and intervention.

Evidence-based interventions are available, but they need to continue to be improved, Chisolm said, especially as more is learned about the effects of cognitive aging. In addition, studies are needed that examine the potential for systematic hearing intervention to influence cognitive, functional and social-emotional status.

Each person with a hearing loss is different, and each will require a different solution. All clinics should conduct speech-in-noise testing and a functional assessment to determine how the hearing loss affects a person's everyday life, Chisolm said; clinics should not just use audiograms. Thresholds are important, but they are "not the be all and end all." Hearing rehabilitative devices and services are usually not covered by insurance, and Chisolm urged that this issue be addressed. Well-controlled studies of both technical and nontechnical interventions could demonstrate the cost-effectiveness and value of interventions.

Finally, Chisolm pointed to an overemphasis on devices rather than comprehensive integrated hearing rehabilitation for older individuals. This workshop could help "change the landscape," she said, so that people can learn to live well with hearing loss as a part of healthy aging.

THE CURRENT U.S. HEARING HEALTH CARE MODEL

Margaret I. Wallhagen
University of California, San Francisco

Hearing loss is seen by many to be a communication disorder, but it may have much more wide-ranging consequences. It could increase the risk of falls and injuries, lead to increased functional limitation and subsequent disability, and reduce one's activity and participation, leading to decreased quality of life. People who have hearing loss often delay seeking hearing health care. Aspects of the hearing health care system help explain why this is and how it might be changed, said Margaret Wallhagen, professor of gerontological nursing at the University of California, San Francisco.

Many stakeholders are involved in the hearing health care system, including the following:

- Consumers and their support associations
- Health care providers
- Hearing health care providers
- Industries and manufacturers
- Centers for Medicare & Medicaid Services (CMS)
- Other health care payers
- Legislators and other policy makers
- Public health professionals

The *Healthy People 2020* goals for hearing and other sensory or communication disorders[2] include the following:

- ENT-VSL-3: Increase the proportion of persons with hearing impairments who have ever used a hearing aid or assistive listening devices or who have cochlear implants

---

[2] See http://www.healthypeople.gov/2020/topicsobjectives2020 (accessed July 8, 2014) for a full listing of objectives. Also, refer to Chapter 7 of this summary for more on *Healthy People 2020*.

- ENT-VSL-4: Increase the proportion of persons who have had a hearing examination on schedule
- ENT-VSL-6: Increase the use of hearing protection devices

Far too few health care providers know about these goals, said Wallhagen.

Medicare uses three conditions to determine coverage: does a service fall within the defined Medicare benefit category, is it reasonable and necessary for diagnosis and treatment, and is it not statutorily excluded for coverage. Unfortunately Medicare has a statutory exclusionary clause prohibiting payment under Part A or Part B "for any expenses incurred for items or services [for] hearing aids or examinations." Said Wallhagen, "I always tell my students, 'We will give you a new heart, but we won't be able to give you glasses, dentures, or hearing aids.'" Various legislators have tried to change the exclusionary clause in Medicaid prohibiting reimbursement for hearing aids, but these efforts have yet to yield results.

The hearing health care system can roughly be characterized as progressing from the consumer to the primary care provider or other provider to the hearing health care specialist. A consumer can go directly to a hearing health care specialist, but referrals are needed to obtain coverage of the assessment by the audiologist.

Consumers tend to attribute hearing loss to normal aging, to be unaware of the extent of hearing loss because of slow onset, to not accord hearing loss a high priority, and to be very concerned about cost. Stigma can also be a factor with hearing loss, especially when the media advertise hearing aids that are "so small no one will know," as Wallhagen put it. A better message would be that people with hearing loss really want to hear what others are saying.

Providers in the primary care setting could overcome many of the barriers to accessing good hearing health care. Yet most do not screen for, pay much attention to, or even know much about hearing loss. According to the U.S. Preventive Services Task Force, between 40 and 86 percent of health care providers admitted they did not screen routinely, with barriers noted including a lack of time, the perception that there are more pressing clinical issues, and a lack of reimbursement (Chou et al., 2011). In an interview of 91 patients conducted by Wallhagen and her colleague, 85 percent of those who had good recall of a clinical encounter said that their practitioners never talked to them about having a hearing screening unless the patient specifically mentioned a hearing problem (Wallhagen and Pettengill, 2008). "We had one woman who kept talking about the fact that she went to see her practitioner who knew she had hearing loss, and [the practitioner] looked in her ears and said, 'They are very nice and clean.' Another [asked his practitioner], 'My wife thinks I have hearing loss,' and the practitioner said that wives say that. Needless to say, the wife was not happy."

This lack of screening is a major problem, Wallhagen said. It was reinforced by the U.S. Preventive Services Task Force, which concluded that "the current evidence is insufficient to assess the balance of benefits and harms of screening for hearing loss in asymptomatic adults aged 50 years or older" (USPSTF, 2012). What is needed from their perspective, Wallhagen stated, is additional research to gain an understanding of the effects of screening compared with no screening on health outcomes and to confirm the benefits of treatment under conditions likely to be encountered in most primary care settings.

The Hearing Health Care System

Once a person is referred for hearing health care, they enter what can be a very confusing system, Wallhagen said. Hearing health care specialists are far from a unified whole. Audiologists may have a Ph.D. or be a doctor of audiology, because that is the requirement for entry into practice. Other practitioners include speech-language pathologists, otolaryngologists (ENT physicians), and hearing instrument specialists (hearing aid dispensers). Some of these categories overlap, and practitioners offer different services to different patients. Specialists and their corresponding professional associations can also disagree among themselves about the types of services practitioners should offer, how services should be reimbursed, and the ways services are accessed by patients. Furthermore, the tension among specialists "is getting larger," said Wallhagen, "because of the new models that are coming out and the various challenges they are facing in terms of their own practices."

The ways in which services are charged also are changing. Many audiologists are arguing that costs should be unbundled because the cost of a hearing aid is not really the cost of the hearing aid by itself but the cost of the hearing aid plus that of surrounding services. Medicaid provisions are also a consideration, though coverage is very state specific and more services are covered for children than for older adults. One model that might be useful, said Wallhagen, is the national Program of All-Inclusive Care for the Elderly (PACE), a model of care which includes integrated medical and social services. The PACE model is based on the On Lok Senior Health Services model started in San Francisco, California, in the early 1970s.[3] Such programs could deal with a patient's greatest needs, including hearing, without worrying about reimbursement issues.

The bottom line, said Wallhagen, is that the hearing health care system

---

[3] See more about the PACE program at www.npaonline.org (accessed May 9, 2014).

is not well coordinated at most levels. Currently it consists more of a menu of offerings, with access restricted by the lack of coverage by Medicare and other insurance companies, consumer beliefs about hearing loss, the cost of hearing aids as currently sold, and a lack of screening and referrals by primary care physicians. Most health care practitioners receive little education around hearing loss. And those involved more directly with issues of hearing loss have a wide range of views about payment strategies that will support their practices and professions.

Wallhagen called for studies that would generate data on the benefits of primary screening and the effectiveness of hearing aids on outcomes and would evaluate models of care that may be targeted to individuals with varying levels of hearing loss. In addition, she said, programs are needed that address the following goals:

- Inform older adults about hearing loss, available options, and how to be educated consumers when seeking treatment;
- Educate health care practitioners (including physicians, nurses, and physician assistants) about hearing loss and available resources; and
- Continue to emphasize that hearing loss is a public health issue.

Screening is particularly an issue in low-income communities, said Wallhagen, where practitioners are often reluctant to screen patients because of the difficulty patients would have in getting hearing devices. In such settings, health care practitioners could at least make patients with hearing loss aware of the communications issues they face and the kinds of devices that could help them stay engaged.

AN INTERNATIONAL PERSPECTIVE

Nikolai Bisgaard
GN ReSound A/S

The six leading hearing aid manufacturers—Oticon, Phonak, ReSound, Siemens, Starkey, and Widex—account for more than 85 percent of the world market, according to Nikolai Bisgaard, vice president of intellectual property rights and industry relations at GN ReSound A/S. All are represented in the European Hearing Instrument Manufacturers Association (EHIMA). This association has standing committees that deal with such issues as standardization and market development. The latter committee, which Bisgaard chairs, seeks to develop and grow the size of the market. For example, its Hear-It website (www.hear-it.org) has been operating for a decade and has been translated into six languages.

The world market for hearing aids in 2012 was about 10.7 million units, Bisgaard said, with a total wholesale revenue of around $5 billion. It is not a huge industry, he added, and, with a steady growth rate of about 2 percent per year, will grow slowly, given current trends. Europe is the largest current market, followed by North America, Asia, and the rest of the world, respectively.

Objective data about the use of hearing aids are generally unavailable, said Bisgaard, but he said estimates based on the number of units sold suggest that about 20 percent of the adult population with hearing impairments in the United States and Europe use hearing aids, falling to 11 percent in Japan, 6 percent in Russia, 2 percent in China, and less than 1 percent in India. Hearing care is clearly associated with a higher standard of living. "If you live in a developing country and get some money, hearing aids are not the first thing you think about," said Bisgaard. "You would rather have cell phones, refrigerators, TV sets, and the like."

The use of hearing aids varies widely within Europe, Bisgaard observed, from a high of 56 percent of the hearing-impaired adult population in Denmark to single digits in many countries of southern and eastern Europe. The general standard of living among countries accounts for some of these differences, he said, but so do differences in accessibility to hearing health care, subsidy levels, and general historical factors. "Some countries have had free hearing aids for ages. Other countries introduced it recently, and some don't have anything of the sort."

The delivery systems for hearing health care also differ within Europe. High-use areas are characterized by public hospitals with audiology departments, Bisgaard observed. Many of these areas offer free, good-quality hearing aids for all citizens with a recognized hearing loss, though some may only partially cover hearing aids purchased from a private dispenser. In Denmark, for example, patients receive vouchers from the government that will cover the cost of a hearing aid with basic features from a private dispenser. The Netherlands offers a 75 percent refund from the public health care system for a hearing aid from a private dispenser. In the United Kingdom, the government does not offer a subsidy to private dispensers.

The central European model is more insurance based, Bisgaard noted, though people are required to carry insurance. This insurance will cover 10 to 20 percent of the best possible hearing aids. As in high-use areas, patients need to see an ENT physician, who will refer them to a hearing aid dispenser. The ENT physician then verifies the results before the insurance money is released. The southern European model has minimal public support and features private dispensing, reasonable accessibility, and partial public coverage of costs for challenged groups. In eastern Europe, public support tends to be even more limited, and accessibility tends to be low.

In 2007 a French initiative created a standard for services offered by hearing aid professionals, which was adopted as a European standard in 2010 (CEN, 2010). This EN 15927 standard establishes requirements for education, facilities, equipment, the fitting process, and quality management systems. Its scope is for typical age-related losses, and it acknowledges that children, cochlear implants, and multiple disabilities require further efforts.

A country-by-country analysis by Bisgaard revealed that subsidies for hearing health care and hearing devices increase hearing aid use. Bisgaard described the case of Denmark, which in 1960 introduced free hearing aids for anyone in need; the aids were provided by audiology clinics at public hospitals. Each clinic had a wide choice of products from preapproved suppliers. In 2000 the coverage was among the best in the world, at around 25 percent. Waiting lists for the eighteen auditory clinics were normally from 3 to 8 months, however. In 2001 a new system opened up for private dispensing, with vouchers that allowed for a hearing aid with basic features for fitting in private shops instead of hospital clinics. The client could choose to upgrade to products with more advanced features for private payment. Many private dispensers were established, resulting in a considerable drain of staff from public clinics and even longer waiting lists. Meanwhile, advertising in newspapers and on television exploded. In response, the total market grew by 80 percent over 11 years. Today, more people get hearing aids through private sources than public ones, and a recent survey has shown that people on average are happier with the service they receive in the private outlets than in public clinics, said Bisgaard.

Increased accessibility and visibility of hearing aids increase their use, Bisgaard suggested. Furthermore, when more people have hearing aids, it reduces the stigma surrounding their use. "You will not have the feeling that it is something special. This is not evidence or science. It is just my personal reflection on what we have seen happen here. It has accelerated in Denmark partly because you see more people with hearing aids, and you think they look okay with it." Hearing aids are also less obtrusive and function better than they did 10 years ago, both of which, Bisgaard asserted, have helped increase coverage.

Bisgaard added that early interventions could pay immense social dividends by allowing older people to remain at work and contribute to society in other ways. People might think that hearing is not affecting their jobs or their relations with others, but when a large sample was interviewed about their conditions at work, those with hearing loss reported far more difficulties even when they said that their hearing was not a factor at work. Furthermore, when people come in to get a hearing aid after many years of denial, they tend to have much more difficulty adapting to a hearing device than people who come in when they begin to have problems.

Bisgaard also pointed to some challenges on the horizon. As the population ages, the overall total cost for hearing devices will increase, which has already led to some pushback from insurance companies and public systems. At the same time, hearing aids are getting better every year and becoming increasingly attractive, so more people want to use them. Supplying large segments of a population with hearing devices can be expensive, Bisgaard pointed out. The populations of some countries may be willing to pay for such services through taxes and other means, whereas others may not. "This is an equation that is not easy to solve."

Subsidies could be reduced and patients differentiated, Bisgaard observed. For example, a child with a hearing loss may receive better services than an older adult. The bundling of services into hearing aids might also change, though this is a "delicate matter," Bisgaard said. But "it is inevitable that it is going to come up some day and that we need to work with that dimension." People are accustomed to paying for part of their dental and vision services, Bisgaard concluded, and they will likely need to do so with hearing as well, though subsidies will improve their likelihood of moving forward.

5

Hearing Technologies

Technologies are changing even faster than the hearing health care system is, and in many ways technologies are driving changes in that system. Four speakers at the workshop provided both wide-angle and more narrowly focused perspectives on these changes, including the regulation, standardization, and assessment of technologies.

A TECHNOLOGY OVERVIEW

Cynthia Compton-Conley
Compton-Conley Consulting

As Cynthia Compton-Conley, chief executive officer of Compton-Conley Consulting, described in an overview of hearing technologies, a wide variety of hearing instruments and hearing assistance technologies are available for people with mild to profound hearing loss (see Figure 5-1). All have become more powerful and sophisticated over time.

Nevertheless, hearing aids and implants do have limitations. First, when microphones are worn on the head, speech understanding is negatively influenced by room acoustics. The target signal, whether speech or music, can become too soft, can be covered up (masked) by noise, and can be smeared by reverberation. Often a combination of these deleterious effects occurs. Directional microphones can improve understanding in some settings, but not in all.

Second, some of the technologies do not work for media such as iPods or telephones. For example, hearing aids and implants need additional ac-

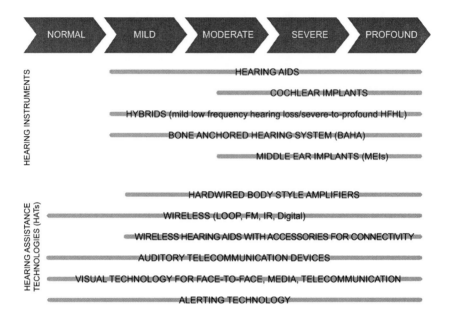

FIGURE 5-1 Range of types of hearing instruments and hearing-assistance technologies available for people with normal hearing to profound hearing losses.
NOTE: FM = frequency modulation; HFHL = high frequency hearing loss; IR = infrared.
SOURCE: Reprinted with permission, Cynthia Compton-Conley © 2013.

cessories to provide private listening to music with an MP3 player. In addition, some hearing aids, if held near certain cell phones, will buzz, requiring additional technologies to enhance communication.

Finally, technologies do not always warn people about convenience sounds, security sounds, or other cues. In the past, said Compton-Conley, people only had one ringtone. Now they may have 10 ringtones plus many other sounds alerting them to things that need to be heard or done.

Communication Needs

All people have four receptive communication needs, Compton-Conley said—face-to-face, media, telecommunications, and alerting—and all four of these needs must be met in various venues of a person's life, whether at home, work, school, play, or volunteer sites. In each venue, an existing technology may need a slight modification, or an entirely different technology may be needed.

One approach to deal with these shifting demands is through a partnership between personal hearing instruments and hearing assistance technologies, said Compton-Conley. Such partnerships can extend the improvement in communication that modern hearing aids and implants make possible. These approaches can be classified into the categories of personal versus private, portable versus stationary, and hardwired versus wireless. With face-to-face communications or the reception of media, for instance, a microphone or other device can pick up a signal and transmit the signal to a receiver that is coupled to a hearing aid or implant, which Compton-Conley described as "binoculars for the ears." An example is the common portable FM system, in which a microphone/transmitter picks up a signal and transmits it wirelessly to a receiver coupled to a hearing aid, implant, or set of headphones. The selection of coupling depends on the person and situation and would need to be determined through a needs assessment process.

This approach has many different applications and associated technologies. For example, a television may connect wirelessly to a Bluetooth transceiver that then sends the signal wirelessly to a hearing device. Or a signal may travel directly through a wireless connection from a lapel microphone or television to a hearing aid. Such systems can also be used in the workplace, though things can become complicated if more than one employee has a hearing loss and each uses a different wireless hearing aid system, Compton-Conley noted. In some settings where it is important that a signal not leave the room, infrared or encrypted FM transmission can be used.

Compton-Conley also described induction loops, which can be used in many settings. A loop of wire goes all the way around a room and is connected to an amplifier that is plugged into a television or other signal source. As soon as a person walks into the room, a signal is sent to a telecoil inside a hearing aid or implant. "You can loop a table, a chair, an office. This room [where the workshop was held] was looped." FM transmitters are also used in public places such as theaters or schools to send signals to hearing devices. Under the Americans with Disabilities Act (ADA), for example, theaters and other public venues are required to have acoustic and inductive coupling.

These systems are far from perfect, Compton-Conley said. People going into a theater hand over a driver's license and are then given a receiver with a neck loop when they really wanted one with earphones. Patrons may also discover that the receiver is dead, so the manager needs to find a new battery. The signal may be intermittent or the volume control broken. "The manager says, 'I don't know what to tell you. We are in compliance. We are following the law.' He gives you your money back, he gives you your ID back. [But] you are really unhappy."

Then again, such systems can work perfectly, as in the case of a venue that has been looped according to the standards of the International Electrotechnical Commission. In this case, if the listener's telecoils are perfectly programmed, then all the listener needs to do is purchase the ticket, walk inside the venue, and flip the hearing aid to telecoil (or MT [for microphone and telecoil]); the listener can then enjoy the show.

A new technology known as frequency-hopping spread spectrum is portable and has the same coupling options as FM. It can be used for one-way or two-way communication and for small-group or large-group settings. "I did a setup one time where there was a Spanish-speaking tour guide speaking to a hard-of-hearing Spanish-to-English interpreter to a group of hard-of-hearing and normal-hearing people who needed to talk back to the tour guide through the interpreter," Compton-Conley said. What is needed is to assess the needs of the group and set up rules of communication. "It is a mix of technology and training," she noted. "You can't solve problems with just technology. People have to know how to use it."

These many options can seem confusing, Compton-Conley acknowledged, and they can be even more confusing to older people. Systems can be incompatible, and each person's system must be adjusted to achieve the best signal. Systems requiring receivers also need to be maintained, and hearing aid or implant users need telecoils to access public systems.

Telephones and Alerting Devices

Many different systems also exist to access phones and other telecommunications systems, including add-on amplifiers, hands-free interfaces, and speech-to-text services. In addition to many varieties of hardwired and wireless systems, live captioning is available for phones or teleconferences either by itself or in addition to auditory input. Some people use automatic voicemail transcription services so that voicemail is received as a text or an e-mail. Specialty professional devices such as amplified or visual stethoscopes are also available.

Finally, Compton-Conley covered alerting devices for homes, offices, and public areas, including alarm clocks, doorbells, phones, crying babies, appliance alerts, weather alerts, motion detectors, smoke alarms, and security alarms. These systems, too, can be hardwired or wireless, and they can use an auditory signal, a tactile signal, or both. For example, Compton-Conley once set up a pressure mat for a woman with Alzheimer's disease so that if she walked out of her bedroom in the middle of the night, the bed of her severely hard-of-hearing daughter and son-in-law would shake. Similarly, a gateway (transceiver) device worn at the waist can pick up a signal from an alerting device and then cause a hearing aid to beep as well as flash lights around the home.

Fire safety is a particular concern, given that individuals older than age 65 have a fire death rate more than twice the national average. Most current smoke detectors have peak sounds at about 3100 hertz, which is right where many older people have hearing loss. When people are asleep, the alerting signal needs to be about 40 dB louder than when they are awake, Compton-Conley said. Also, many people with hearing loss incorrectly assume that they will be able to hear a smoke detector because they can hear it when they test it. "If you are in a deep sleep, on medication, are sleep deprived, or [have your head] under your pillow, and your smoke detector is behind a closed door, you might not hear it."[1] "Fire safety alerting systems for individuals with hearing impairment need to be recommended more often," she said.

Disruptive Technologies

Companies are beginning to explore disruptive technologies that could change the paradigm, Compton-Conley reported. First-generation devices are being developed that can stream virtually any signal from a smart phone to wireless hearing aids. People would still need telecoils for large public areas, but eventually signals could be available from such areas that go directly to phones and then to a hearing aid, avoiding receiver maintenance and coupling issues.

Another disruptive technology would be a chip built into hearing aids that could convert signals from any model of hearing enhancement device. Similar sorts of universal design technologies could meet all four hearing needs while also providing hearing protection. Research is under way on self-fitting hearing aids that measure hearing thresholds, create an on-the-fly prescription, and fine-tune a device over time to meet a person's listening needs. And smartphones could eventually be used as hardwired universal hearing enhancement devices.

The critical question, said Compton-Conley, is what consumers want and need and how best to meet those needs. One obvious thing they want is full communication access for a lifetime, which requires a holistic needs assessment process, including careful assessment of residual hearing using best practices, speech, and noise testing. This assessment process would look at a person's health, situation, finances, and comfort with technology which would yield a customized set of technologies and training that are verified and validated. "People make the mistake of jumping into the technology before they analyze the needs," said Compton-Conley. "Or they analyze the needs, they recommend the technology, and they don't program the telecoil, for example. This needs to stop."

Compton-Conley concluded with several ideas that she said should be

---

[1] Specific information related to fire safety may be found at www.soundstrategy.com/tutorials/how-alerting-technology-can-keep-you-and-your-family-safe-and-add-convenience-your-life (accessed February 26, 2014).

adopted to meet existing challenges. First, she said a required sequence of coursework for hearing health care providers is needed that is standardized across training programs and focused on best practices, along with more rigorous accreditation. She also recommended an open-platform universal design that provides simplified selection and fitting, easier consumer access, and minimal maintenance for venues; instructional applications for personal and public access, including an assistive listening devices locator; and a massive informational campaign, including a checklist for consumers. She added that continued research and development is needed on self-fitting, self-adjustable, open-platform devices. Finally, Compton-Conley supported an open market for both prescribed and nonprescribed hearing enhancement products.

In conclusion, Compton-Conley recalled an elderly patient who came in with his son and his wife of more than 60 years. He had brain stem injuries due to repeated strokes, and hearing aids were not an option. He was also in a wheelchair and had visual problems, so captioning was not an option for him. During the case history, he was unresponsive, so Compton-Conley gave him a set of earphones attached to an FM receiver. When she talked into the microphone connected to her own FM transmitter, Compton-Conley said, the patient "perked up." She asked him what he had for breakfast, and he answered with animated detail. Compton-Conley said his wife and son were amazed. The man lived 5 more years and was able to communicate easily with his wife, son, and extended family. He was also able to listen to the television, as well as hear his wife, by using the FM receiver equipped with a direct plug-in to the television and a remote microphone placed on the table between him and his wife. Compton-Conley said this case illustrates the importance of assessing a person's needs first and then applying appropriate technology and training. It also points out that a range of technologies is available to provide communication access.

CURRENT FDA STANDARDS

Eric A. Mann
U.S. Food and Drug Administration

The U.S. Food and Drug Administration (FDA) derives its regulatory authority to oversee the safety and effectiveness of medical devices from the Food, Drug, and Cosmetic Act, which specifies in section 201 that a medical device is intended to diagnose, cure, mitigate, treat, or prevent a disease or condition, or is intended to affect the structure or function of the body, and does not achieve its intended use through chemical action or metabolism. This is a very broad definition, said Eric Mann, clinical deputy director for the Division of Ophthalmic and Ear, Nose, and Throat Devices in the Center for Devices and Radiological Health at the FDA, but "it does draw a bright line between things that are medical devices and those that aren't." By this definition, a hearing aid is clearly a medical device. In contrast, a personal sound amplification product (PSAP), in the FDA's view, is a product meant to be used by normally hearing people under certain listening conditions. Thus, the FDA distinguishes between a hearing aid, which treats hearing-impaired consumers of any degree, and a PSAP, which is for normally hearing individuals. The FDA recently updated a guidance document in draft form to clarify the types of claims that would be associated with hearing aids and with PSAPs.

Because a huge range of devices fall under its purview, from tongue depressors to pacemakers, the FDA applies a risk-based classification in which the regulatory requirements are matched to the risk posed by the device. Class I devices are considered low risk; Class II, moderate risk; and Class III, high risk. For Class I devices, baselines levels of regulatory requirements that apply across all device types are intended to ensure the safety and effectiveness of the device. For Class II devices, additional special controls are needed, such as a performance standard, points that need to be addressed in a premarket submission, or a postmarket surveillance requirement such as a registry or a device-tracking mechanism. Class III devices must undergo a premarket approval process, which generally requires a well-designed clinical study and information on manufacturing.

Different kinds of hearing devices fit into different categories. A typical air conduction hearing aid is considered a low-risk Class I device. Class II devices include such devices as bone-conduction hearing aids, bone-anchored hearing aids, and tinnitus maskers. Wireless air conduction hearing aids can also be Class II devices, not because of risks from the hearing aid but because of the regulatory controls needed to ensure their effectiveness given wireless interference and other issues. Class III auditory devices include technologies such as cochlear implants, implantable middle ear hearing devices, and auditory brain stem implants.

Mann focused most of his remarks on Class I devices, because they were the focus of the workshop. For these devices, the FDA has determined that general controls in and of themselves are sufficient to ensure safety and effectiveness. General controls include the following:

- The prohibition of adulterated or misbranded devices so that labeling is not false or misleading
- The use of good manufacturing practices
- Registration of manufacturing facilities and listing of device types
- Record-keeping requirements
- Provisions for repair, replacement, and refund (though these rarely come into play, said Mann)

When the medical device amendments were first enacted in 1976, there was a requirement for premarket notification, also known as a 510(k), for Class I devices. Since the late 1990s, most Class I devices have been exempt from that requirement for premarket notification. Thus, as long as they comply with the general controls, the manufacturers of air conduction hearing aids would not have to submit a premarket application to the FDA. The exceptions, said Mann, would be if a fundamental change in technology to the hearing aid occurred or if the hearing aid were being indicated for a new population, which would exceed the limitations of the exemption and would require a 510(k).

Provisions for Hearing Aids

A handful of devices at the FDA have separate regulations to ensure their safety and effectiveness, and hearing aids are among those devices. One regulation governs labeling (21 CFR 801.420); another governs the conditions for sale (21 CFR 801.421).

For labeling, the regulations require hearing aid manufacturers to develop a user instructional brochure. The regulation outlines the content of that brochure, requiring, for example, well-defined instructions for use and notification that the hearing aid will not restore normal hearing. A "Warning to Hearing Aid Dispensers" lists what are often referred to as "red flag signs and symptoms," such as draining from the ear or asymmetric hearing loss. An "Important Notice for Prospective Hearing Aid Users" describes the conditions for sale and the need for a medical evaluation. A technical performance data section is also required as defined by a standard from the American National Standards Institute (ANSI).

For the conditions for sale, the regulations require a medical evaluation by a licensed physician within the preceding 6 months of dispensing a hearing aid. A waiver of the medical evaluation is possible for users more than 18 years of age as long as the patient signs a statement acknowledging that a medical evaluation is in his or her best health interest. The dispenser may not encourage the waiver, and the dispenser must afford patients an opportunity to review the user instructional brochure. Record-keeping requirements for 3 years are also specified.

Both of these regulations were the product of recommendations from an interdepartmental task force and U.S. Senate hearings that were held in the mid-1970s to look into the suboptimal diagnosis and treatment of hearing disorders prior to dispensing a hearing aid, as well as the marketing of hearing aids to vulnerable individuals who did not need them. The regulations are based not on safety issues with the hearing aid but on recognizing medically and surgically treatable causes of hearing loss and providing optimal hearing health care for patients, said Mann.

Discussion

As Mann said, if a PSAP were to make claims about treating hearing-impaired individuals, then it crosses the line and meets the definition of a medical device. The FDA could then take enforcement action to require conformance with the medical device regulations, including the specific regulations for hearing aids.

Frank Lin pointed out that PSAPs are linked with issues of access. Many people do not have enough money to buy a hearing aid. Access to some type of rudimentary PSAP device could improve their lives. "In the field of audiology and acoustic sciences, there is always the pursuit of perfection. We want the absolute best." But often the best is not necessary, Lin observed. "The way we approach hearing health care right now is that you either have everything or you have nothing." The gap between a PSAP and a hearing aid is essentially narrowing to nothing, he said. "It is how you market it and how you label it." Lin argued that something is better than nothing. "My question is, what can we do, from a regulatory point of view, to make access to such devices possible?"

Mann responded that the FDA does not distinguish between a rudimentary hearing aid and a more advanced hearing aid. The regulations define a hearing aid as a wearable instrument that is intended for hearing-impaired individuals. He also pointed out, however, that the regulations are not incompatible with a direct-to-consumer marketing model, as long as the labeling requirements are met and a waiver is signed. "We have been fairly liberal in terms of interpreting this," he said. "As long as the patient has the opportunity to review the user instructional brochure, and as long as the record-keeping requirements are complied with, a manufacturer can directly market to a consumer." Many people are using these waivers, he acknowledged, but signing the waiver could be of some benefit to patients by informing them of conditions that could be treatable. If a hearing aid then does not solve their problem, or if they encounter progression of their hearing loss, they may be more likely to see a physician as a result of that counseling process. "It is a complicated issue," he said. "We are willing to listen to different perspectives on this. There certainly is a process—kind of a cumbersome one—to change regulations, but it exists."

Still, he also noted that hearing aids are different from reading glasses, where it is much easier for individuals to self-diagnose their conditions and to decide whether magnifying eyeglasses are an appropriate solution for their particular health situation. Hearing loss can result from a large variety of serious health conditions that could potentially be detected by a medical evaluation, Mann said.

WIRELESS STANDARDS

Stephen Berger
TEM Consulting

Standards are tools that can serve a variety of purposes, said Stephen Berger, president of TEM Consulting:

- They can be multiparty contracts.
- They can be vehicles for knowledge transfer.
- They can be specifications to ensure different kinds of interoperability.
- They are a vehicle for facilitating conformity assessment and management.
- They can be a tool for technology planning.

Berger described each of these purposes in turn.

Multiparty Contracts

As an example of a multiparty contract, Berger cited the ANSI C63.19 standard governing the compatibility of hearing aids with mobile phones. The standard, on which work started in 1996, is mandated by the Federal Communications Commission and recognized by the FDA. "In general, we have been successful," said Berger. "Obviously, we didn't get it perfect out of the box. We are on standard version four and are actively talking about what we might need to do in version five. Also, in both industries, technology has changed."

One lesson learned from this experience is that consensus is almost impossible when costs and consequences are not aligned. It is not unusual to encounter a circumstance where if one industry were to pay a little more, another industry would benefit. But "how are you going to make that happen?" asked Berger. "It is not easy." At the beginning of the development of the C63.19 standard, both industries, which are quite different, accused the other of being the source of the problem. The impasse was broken when one of the phone companies sent several engineers to a hearing aid chip manufacturer to show how to make a chip immune from interference. This gave the chip manufacturer and any phone company that bought the chips a way to differentiate their products from those of their competitors. "All of a sudden, market forces started kicking in," said Berger. "We got a consensus and finished the standard."

Knowledge Transfer

This process created a lot of knowledge transfer, said Berger. Bodies of experts exchanged knowledge and sought to understand each other's landscape enough to find consensus solutions. That is happening today in the hearing aid industry as the move to digital technologies shifts attention from simply raising the volume of sounds to issues of signal quality. Similarly, the standard for radio frequency interference is now based on the amount of interference created in the hearing aid rather than just the amount of potential interference from radio frequency sources.

Interoperability

Different kinds of interoperability exist. One is simply that if two devices are close together, they do not interfere with each other's operation. Another is that two devices may rely on different equipment, but their measures and outputs mean the same thing. A third is that units from different vendors work with each other, either for core functions or for all functions. Achieving interoperability can have both positive and negative effects, said Berger. For example, bringing people together to create interoperability can have the effect of stifling innovation.

An effective feedback system is almost always necessary to create interoperability, Berger said. If laboratories do not test a device properly, even a wonderful standard will not produce a desired outcome. Similarly, market experiences typically need to feed back into a standard to get the outcomes sought by the standard.

Conformity Assessment and Management

Conformity assessment and management help ensure that products meet their specifications in actual use. The people who wrote a standard know what they had in mind, but the standard needs to be translated to ensure that requirements lead to the right outcomes. If this is done properly, good products get through, and those that are below par get returned for further work. In this way, standards can also facilitate market forces. When consumers do not know how to distinguish an excellent product from a poorly designed product, they cannot make informed choices.

Technology Planning

Finally, standards further technology planning by helping to keep industries synchronized, he said. Thus, as the cell phone industry moves to the fourth generation, standards enable the hearing aid industry to remain synced with changes in cell phones. Also, different technologies require different metrics, as demonstrated by the history of audio quality standards. And a particularly difficult challenge is how to "end-of-life" a technology and move to a better solution, said Berger. "How do we give incentives for people to move to a new and potentially much better solution while not leaving people isolated and orphaned with what had been the previous solution? It is something we need to map out, or else our regulations end up becoming anti-innovative, which is not where we want to be."

Interesting work is going on in understanding the relational links between seemingly unrelated areas, Berger noted. The task is to map and then manage the complex ontology surrounding hearing loss. "Most of what we have been talking about is trying to understand what is this ontology that we are all working at? What are the dynamics? What are the relational links? How do we manage it to get to a better future?" Understanding the types of innovation would shed light on this ontology. For example, are innovations disruptive, sustaining, or obstructive? What are both the intended and unintended consequences of innovation?

Standards are not a panacea, Berger asserted. They are "great when they are the right tool for the job. They are lousy when they are mismatched or just a feel-good exercise." Standards can have the effect of suppressing innovation, and regulators and standards developers need to minimize that possibility. Therefore, both standards and regulations must focus on the required outcomes while being slow to dictate methods for achieving those outcomes. Another challenge is to move from a consensus that has been right for the past to one that is right for the future. Still, standards can also document a multiparty consensus, and "when they do that well, they can be really powerful," Berger concluded.

HEALTH TECHNOLOGY ASSESSMENT: ROLE IN TECHNOLOGY DEVELOPMENT AND USE

Fiona A. Miller
University of Toronto

Health technology assessment (HTA) is a field of applied policy analysis designed to support decisions about payment for health technologies, including drugs, devices, diagnostics, procedures, and even different ways of organizing health care. It is "an evidence-informed and a value-laden enterprise that plays an important and growing role in determining what kinds of technologies and services will be available for patients within health care systems," said Fiona Miller, associate professor of health policy at the University of Toronto's Institute of Health Policy, Management, and Evaluation. It is also increasingly being used to support technology development.

Miller pointed out that, in modern health care systems, health care is not primarily financed through payments by users for their own care. Rather, health care is primarily financed through collective payment mechanisms, whether public or private. The United States is not an exception to this observation. For example, out-of-pocket expenditures on care as a percentage of total health expenditures is actually lower in the United States than in Canada, even though Canada has a single-payer system. "The vast majority of health care is provided collectively," said Miller. "We pay for each other's care, not so much for our own."

Of course, the coverage of hearing aids and other hearing-related technologies, as pointed out by other speakers, varies. The province where Miller lives provides substantial coverage of these technologies, whereas coverage is much more limited in the United States. These coverage provisions can be important, she pointed out, because small things can have a major impact on healthy aging. As people age, hips, knees, and hearts are important, but so is support for living at home, transportation, and meals, said Miller. Supports for simple things like clearing the snow or picking up groceries can help older adults to avoid a fall and the subsequent need for long-term or rehabilitative care. "These are the types of small things that enable people to age healthfully."

Hearing aids are among the small things that matter, Miller argued. People with chronic and debilitating conditions are by far the largest source of health care expenditures, but most people can be supported through self-care and low levels of supportive care. To the extent that hearing technologies can support healthy aging and avoid the need for higher-cost technologies, they can be an important part of the health assessment conversation.

The Development of the HTA Field

HTA emerged in the United States in the 1970s but is now well developed internationally. The International Network of Agencies for HTA now includes 57 member agencies from 32 countries. In the United States, the Agency for Healthcare Research and Quality is a major supporter and conductor of HTA.

A basic premise of the field is that "newly approved" does not always mean new or improved. Health technology regulations ask whether a technology is safe to have on the market, at least for a specific class of patients. HTA asks different questions: Is technology safe and at least as good as the alternatives in the real world? Also, is it worthwhile to invest in this technology?

Today, HTA has a variable role in health care systems, Miller observed. In some health care systems, it is still fairly detached from coverage. It provides guidance but does not necessarily guide coverage decisions. In other health care systems, it does directly inform coverage. For example, the National Institute for Health and Clinical Excellence (NICE) in the United Kingdom reviews technologies and decides whether they will be provided and covered. Within each Canadian province—each of which essentially has its own health care system—health technology assessment often has a fairly close link to the decision to cover a technology. Sometimes the procedure is even more embedded in decision making. In Canada and some European countries, a movement has gained momentum to locate HTA within a regional health authority or hospital to inform decisions on investments within annual budgets.

Forms of Evidence

HTA involves different kinds of evidence. The most important is clinical evidence, which includes the evidence of *safety and efficacy* that a regulatory authority would demand, as well as evidence of real-world effectiveness and comparative effectiveness. "We want to know how [a new technology] compares to the existing best-case scenario, or at least to another technology or package of services that is being used."

Another form of evidence is *economic*. Because health care is primarily paid for collectively, the question is whether a new technology represents a good use of limited resources, in recognition of the opportunity cost of not investing in the next best alternative. "If you bring in five new technologies that cost X, something has to give." Although the United States has resisted taking this step, said Miller, Canada and most of Europe have been more willing to look at the economic evidence. Value for money, the impact on budgets, and affordability are all relevant issues.

HTA also takes *patient and social values* into account. It looks at patient preferences, health equity, and transparency and clarity in the actions of agencies, which Miller referred to as "accountability for reasonableness." Obviously, it is a "fraught and complex exercise," she said.

HTA Experiments

Historically, HTA has focused "downstream" on the implications of novel technologies for health and health care, assessing whether health technologies warrant adoption; accordingly, HTA has often been seen as a barrier to innovation. Increasingly, however, HTA is looking "upstream" at innovation processes, seeking to support decisions about the design and development of emerging technologies; from this perspective, HTA has a role as a facilitator within productive health innovation systems. Miller described three types of experiments taking place around the world that position HTA as a facilitator of health innovation. In the United Kingdom, for example, the emphasis has been on innovation adoption. Thus, where a technology is seen to merit investment, concerted attention is given to ensuring that it is used equitably and broadly across the appropriate populations.

A second experiment involves harmonization of evidence requirements across HTA agencies or between regulatory agencies and HTA agencies. With hearing aids, for example, would it be possible to align the evidence that regulators want with the evidence needed for HTA? This question has been much discussed in Europe and elsewhere, Miller reported.

A third experiment involves "early" HTA, where technology assessments are conducted early in the development process to inform technology design and provide decision support for industry. Early assessment helps industry to learn sooner whether a technology will meet the expectations of payers: "Fail fast and fail early if you are going to fail," Miller said. In Ontario, for example, an initiative with which Miller is involved, called MaRS EXCITE,[2] seeks to be a single portal for evidence generation and review early in the design and development phase. "We are working with large multinational enterprises, but also small and medium size enterprises, that sometimes have no idea in the design and development phase what they will need to show to justify payment by Ontario's health care system."

CONCLUSION

HTA can play an important role in analyzing the merits of health care investments, Miller concluded. It can provide both a guide and an incentive for supporting technological innovations that will improve health, including technologies relevant to hearing loss.

In response to a question about whether the demands of regulators and HTA agencies for evidence of safety, efficacy, and effectiveness might stifle innovation, Miller pointed out that this is "the classic countervailing powers question." Perhaps a small mom-and-pop shop will not be successful, she said, but the question is, do we want the small mom-and-pop shop to be successful if that means items that did not pass any meaningful regulatory hurdle are on the market? For instance, the pharmaceutical industry no longer has mom-and-pop companies as it did at the end of the nineteenth century. The merger of companies is, in part, a response to the regulatory and HTA environment. These demands reflect the reasonable expectation that innovative health technologies will be safe and effective and will address genuine and important health needs.

---

[2] See http://excite.marsdd.com (accessed February 26, 2014).

6

Innovative Models

As is occurring in other major sectors of society, innovation is reshaping the hearing health care system. New technologies, new ways of delivering hearing health care, new policies, and new ideas about design are changing how people access, use, and pay for hearing devices. This chapter brings together five presentations at the workshop that examined these innovations, which together have the potential to transform how people around the world confront and overcome age-related hearing loss.

THE COMMUNITY HEALTH WORKER MODEL[1]

Prepared by: Nicole Marrone, University of Arizona
Presented by: Theresa Chisolm, University of South Florida

Community health workers are front-line public health workers who are trusted lay members of the community they serve, observed Theresa Chisolm, professor and chair of the Department of Communication Sciences and Disorders at the University of South Florida on behalf of Nicole Marrone, assistant professor and James S. and Dyan Pignatelli/Unisource Clinical Chair in Audiologic Rehabilitation for Adults at the University of Arizona. Community health workers serve as a liaison or intermediary between health or social services and the communities to facilitate individuals' access to services and improve the quality and cultural competence of

---

[1] This presentation was written by and based on the work of Nicole Marrone, but presented on her behalf by Theresa Chisolm.

service delivery. They have many titles, including community health worker, community health advisor or aid, promotora, community health representative, peer health promoter, lay health educator, and patient navigator. Their core competencies include communication, interpersonal skills, service coordination, capacity building, advocacy, teaching, and organizational skills. They provide cultural mediation between communities and health and human services systems, advocate for individual and community needs, and ensure culturally appropriate health education and support.

Community health care workers do not provide clinical care and generally do not hold professional licenses. Nevertheless, they have expertise about the communities they serve because they share cultures and life experience with the members of those communities. They rely on relationships and trust and relate to community members as peers rather than purely as clients or patients.

Previous research has shown that community health care workers can improve access to care, enhance successful chronic disease prevention and management, improve the use of health services (such as reducing the inappropriate use of emergency rooms), help to control costs, and produce a positive return on investment (Ingram et al., 2012; Johnson et al., 2012; Reinschmidt and Chong, 2008; Sabo et al., 2013; Staten et al., 2012; Viswanathan et al., 2009). Research has also demonstrated their effectiveness in addressing health disparities for minority populations, increasing health care utilization, providing culturally competent health education, and advocating for patients' needs (Rosenthal et al., 2010).

Chisolm said that according to Marrone, collaboration with community health workers may be a way to reach people in the community who are otherwise not seeking audiological services. Among Hispanics, for example, far fewer of those who could benefit from hearing aids use themas compared with hearing aid use among the general population. To address this disparity, Nicole Marrone and her colleagues at the University of Arizona are developing a community health worker intervention adapted from her current community-based audiologic rehabilitation program to identify untreated hearing loss in the Hispanic population. Results from that intervention showed that of the adults tested in the community, approximately 76 percent of this urban sample had hearing loss but never had access to care. The program has placed some of these individuals into Spanish-language community-based audiologic rehabilitation groups, which were compared with a group of English-language audiologic rehabilitation participants. Preliminary analyses found that both groups showed improved outcomes in terms of enjoyment of life and daily use of communication strategies even without the use of hearing aids.

As the population ages, all groups will have a growing prevalence of chronic health conditions, including hearing loss. In addition, there are social determinants of health that affect different groups in different ways. Marrone wrote that achieving the goals of *Healthy People 2020* requires a commitment to reduce health inequities across all populations, Chisolm observed.

In collaboration with community providers and community health workers, Marrone is seeking to identify barriers and resources in the community and collaboratively develop an efficacious community health worker intervention in a rural community that is generally underserved and facing great health disparities. This effort includes the development of culturally and linguistically relevant materials and testing of a community health worker model of intervention for older adults with hearing loss. Extensions of this research could evaluate the effectiveness of this model in other geographic regions or with other populations facing health disparities.

TELEAUDIOLOGY

Gabrielle Saunders
National Center for Rehabilitative Auditory Research,
Portland Veterans Affairs Medical Center

Teleaudiology is the delivery of audiology services and information via telecommunications technologies, said Gabrielle Saunders, associate director of the Veterans Affairs (VA) Rehabilitation Research and Development National Center for Rehabilitative Auditory Research in the Portland, Oregon, VA Medical Center. She emphasized that teleaudiology is not a separate subspecialty of audiology. Rather, it is the use of technology as the means to the end of good hearing health.

Telemedicine methodologies can be divided into four categories, Saunders continued. *Store and forward technologies* collect patient data at a remote site and transmit those data to a health care professional to review. *Synchronous or real-time teleaudiology* uses videoconferencing or other means to conduct hearing tests, hearing aid fittings, audiologist-directed real-ear measures, hearing aid counseling, tinnitus management, or other services. *Remote monitoring* involves the patient wearing a device that gathers data that are sent remotely to a health care provider. Finally, *mobile health teleaudiology*, which is the category on which Saunders focused, includes online auditory training programs, tinnitus management, hearing tests, and counseling. It is patient driven and independent of the practitioner. It also raises the largest unknowns for the field because patients are in charge of the technology rather than specialists.

As examples of successful telehealth programs, Saunders mentioned the Alaska Federal Health Care Access Network, established in 1998, which provides services to patients across Alaska at a great cost savings compared with personal services. This program has dramatically decreased wait times for appointments and has produced high patient and provider satisfaction. The VA also has a very active telehealth program that includes audiology services, with more than 1.6 million veterans needing services. This program, too, has produced levels of satisfaction with teleaudiology encounters as high or higher as those of in-person encounters, said Saunders.

Mobile Health

Technology has already made it much easier to access a hearing test, Saunders observed. Online hearing tests, hearing applications, and telephone screening can all test a person's hearing, though each approach raises questions. The first is whether the data are accurate and valid, which at this point is not generally known. "Some of these measures are well designed, and they have been proven to be valid, but not all of them," said Saunders. False negatives can also be a problem if patients are told that they have normal hearing but in fact have a hearing loss. And whether people understand the results from applications and online tests is unclear. In a face-to-face interaction, the patient can ask a question if he or she does not hear or understand what the physician has said, but that generally cannot be done with remote tests.

The bottom-line question, said Saunders, is whether self-conducted tests motivate behavior change. According to a study conducted in Australia, of 193 individuals who failed a telephone-based screening, only 70 sought help; of the 26 who were recommended hearing aids, only 13 obtained them; and of the 13 who obtained hearing aids, only 6 used them more than 4 hours per day (Meyer et al., 2011). These numbers seem very low, Saunders acknowledged, but similar findings are found with face-to-face screening (Yueh et al., 2010). "The issue isn't teleaudiology per se," she said. To overcome these barriers, she noted, the field needs to know more about the attitudes and beliefs underlying hearing health behaviors. In addition, public health messages could be targeted for different age groups to bring awareness of hearing and hearing loss to the whole population, not just to those with increased likelihood of hearing loss.

Assistive Technology

Technology has also made it easier to access hearing assistive technology. Saunders diagrammed some of the distribution systems that exist today for hearing technologies. These include traditional systems (from manufacturer to end user via a private practice), direct distribution (from manufacturer to the end user via a storefront), and semi-direct distribution (wherein a medical doctor and an online hearing aid retailer are involved).

There are also pathways involving online retailers that do or do not also involve local support (e.g., audiologists, other hearing professionals). Most of these pathways involve hearing professionals, but online retailers without local support typically do not. These new models are controversial, she acknowledged, "but they are inevitable, especially with the increased availability of personal sound amplification systems." The field will need to figure out what role audiologists will play if large numbers of consumers start bypassing their services. "We don't know yet, so we need to be conducting that research to find out how these alternative models are going to impact outcomes," Saunders said.

Another way of using technology to acquire hearing assistance is by using a smartphone as a hearing aid. Systematic research will be needed to determine the pros and cons of this approach, Saunders said. Applications and telephone technologies are also available for tinnitus management, with a telephone tinnitus education program for veterans being evaluated in a study at the National Center for Rehabilitative Auditory Research. In addition, technology permits home-based, online computerized auditory training, as discussed earlier in the workshop. Although large randomized studies have not demonstrated benefits from such training, some people in these studies benefited from the training. If those people could be identified in advance, the training could prove useful for at least a subgroup of the population, though the question remains regarding how much they could benefit.

Technology has also spawned online hearing-related support groups, counseling programs, and other online gatherings. Although little work on the value of these groups has been conducted, one study showed positive outcomes (Thorén et al., 2011).

The willingness of patients and providers to use teleaudiology depends on the applications. For example, Saunders stated that recent data show that audiologists are much more willing to use teleaudiology for answering patients' questions or for counseling than to fit a hearing aid or assess its performance, and they are less willing to use teleaudiology with patients receiving their first hearing aid than with experienced hearing aid users. The willingness of patients to use teleaudiology varies, with some being not at all willing to use teleaudiology, but more than half of patients being moderately to extremely willing to use it. Opinions change with experience, such that after using teleaudiology to fine-tune a hearing aid, about two-thirds of 16 patients and 8 audiologists were more positive about the procedure, according to data collected by the company Phonak, Saunders said. Use "can change attitudes," she added, "and that is probably good news for teleaudiology." Nonetheless, the education of clinicians about teleaudiology will need to be approached carefully, she said, to achieve good outcomes.

Teleaudiology raises many other issues, including technology support, contingency plans, privacy concerns, patient expectations, patient health literacy, billing, licensing across jurisdictions, and the integration of tele-audiology into daily practice. Nevertheless, teleaudiology has been demonstrated to provide easy access to hearing health care at many levels, Saunders concluded. It is generally acceptable to patients and clinicians and could open up hearing health care to a broader demographic of individuals. "The question is not will teleaudiology happen—it will," said Saunders, "but how will it happen, and what can we do to ensure it yields positive outcomes for both the patient and the professional?" Answering those questions will require research on usability, effectiveness, and methods for changing hearing health behaviors so that people access the many available options.

THE PRIMARY CARE SETTING[2]

Thomas J. Powers
Lake Havasu City, Arizona

Thomas J. Powers, a family physician from Lake Havasu City, Arizona, helps his patients to "hear life again." Powers has a small practice in Lake Havasu City, which has a year-round population of 52,000. His wife manages the office. He has two receptionists and one medical assistant. He has about 7,600 active patients, 47 percent of whom are between the ages of 45 and 64 and 47 percent of whom are above the age of 65. In a recent 6-month period, he and his coworkers screened 767 patients for hearing problems, tested 107, and fitted 47 with hearing aids. Of those 47 patients, 79 percent were new to hearing aids, and 86 percent reported that they would not have purchased or would have delayed purchasing hearing aids because of their cost. "Certainly the cost is a big issue for these patients," said Powers.

Powers stated that he incorporated hearing testing into his practice because it allowed for more comprehensive care of patients. His medical assistant tests every patient over the age of 40 with a simple hearing test that has four frequencies at 40 dB. In addition, patients fill out a form with a scale from 1 to 10 of how bad their hearing is. If they miss two frequencies and report an 8 or less on the form, Powers recommends that their hearing undergo a more rigorous test. His practice uses an automated pure-tone audiometer with high-quality headphones in a quiet room. Patients fill out a simple form to rule out pathological reasons for hearing loss other than age. If the hearing loss is related to a medical issue—which happens in

---

[2] Data presented in this section were collected by Dr. Powers from his own patient base.

about 20 percent of cases—the patient is referred to an ENT physician or to a hearing clinic in Los Angeles.

If the hearing test demonstrates a significant hearing loss, Powers fits the patient with a demonstration hearing aid in the office. He then assesses comfort and the patient's perception of hearing. "We give them time with it. We invite them to go out to the lobby to see what the TV sounds like. We invite them to go outside to hear what the traffic sounds like, the air, the wind." If the patient decides to purchase a hearing aid, Powers's wife provides information about maintenance and care and goes over the financial part of the transaction. Powers noted that the simplified yet innovative system enables many of his patients to receive hearing health care quickly and efficiently. He added, "we are not going to treat everybody. But we are at least getting a lot of hearing loss taken care of."

The screenings generally are not expected by the patient, Powers observed. They are not asked whether the initial screening can occur because many would say it is not needed. "They don't want to know if they have a hearing loss. They are denying it." The test, which is conducted as part of the vital exams, is simple and takes only a few seconds. Furthermore, the screenings were appreciated by patients, 89 percent of whom were glad or very glad to have their hearing checked and 72 percent of whom probably or definitely would not have had their hearing checked otherwise.

After testing, 44 percent of the patients who needed hearing aids purchased them. Another 13 percent were referred to other physicians, 16 percent said they were not ready for hearing aids, 3 percent insisted that they did not need hearing aids, and 24 percent said that they could not afford hearing aids. The price of their hearing aids was about $1,500 per pair, and 86 percent of those who purchased hearing aids said that they would not have purchased them elsewhere or would have delayed purchasing them elsewhere because of cost. "There is a lot of denial," Powers repeated. He observed that it is often helpful to have a spouse present, as patients will deny any hearing difficulties.

Patients were largely happy with their hearing aids, he said. Seventy-two percent were wearing them 8 to 16 hours per day, 14 percent were wearing them 4 to 8 hours per day, and another 14 percent were wearing them 1 to 4 hours per day. Powers makes sure that the hearing aids are comfortable and working, and his wife handles calls from patients. They even do house visits if a patient is older and cannot come to the office. "They are very satisfied, and they are using them." Powers does not charge for the testing or the fitting. Some patients have a hard time affording the cost, but a credit program is available for those who qualify.

Powers was concerned that the audiologists and the ENT physician in town would react negatively when they heard that he was dispensing hearing aids. But he said that has not been the case. He needs audiologists and

ENT physicians so that he can refer more complicated cases to them. He also pointed out that having an audiologist in the office would be one approach, but interaction with a familiar and trusted primary care physician can be especially powerful for a patient.

Powers noted that many of his patients report that the technology has transformed their lives. "We are making conversations with family easier for them. They are going to movie theatres and understanding speech. They are going to the grocery stores and hearing much better. We are making an improvement in their lives."

The impact on his practice has been minimal, though it does interrupt his schedule somewhat, in that he is seeing hearing aid patients on top of his regular 15-minute-per-patient schedule. But the patients are surprised, grateful, and happy, he said. It also has been rewarding and gratifying to Powers because "it is life-changing to the patients. You put a hearing aid in them and they just wake up." Finally, it is cost-effective.

"We need to get this into family practice residencies," Powers concluded. "We need to get it into primary care. I hope that I am just a stepping block for that."

SOCIAL ENTERPRISE BUSINESS MODELS

David Green
Sound World Solutions

The strategic use of technology, price, and quality can change the competitive landscape in favor of the consumer, said David Green, cofounder of Sound World Solutions. Drawing on his experience with eye care programs around the world, Green described how the combination of affordable technologies with cost-effective and efficient service delivery can achieve the social mission of pricing for affordability and accessibility.

Experiences with Treating Vision Impairment

Around the world, an estimated 285 million people are visually impaired, and 39 million of these are blind in both eyes, said Green. The eye care services Green has provided are self-financed from patient fees and do not depend on any insurance reimbursement system. Where there is tiered pricing, "free" is the lowest price, and revenues are used to subsidize care for those who cannot afford a service or can only pay below cost. This creates not only competition in price-sensitive markets but entirely new ecosystems with markedly reduced costs.

Cataracts are the main cause of blindness and have been the main emphasis of Green's efforts. He has helped more than 300 programs, which together perform about 1 million surgeries per year, become self-financing. One of the best known is Aravind Eye Hospital in India, which provides more than 370,000 surgeries per year. Green described the hospital's model where 51 percent of patients get service either for free or below cost. The remainder pay above cost, and the margin is used to cross-subsidize care. Even with this cross-subsidization, Aravind in 2012 was able to make a 33 percent margin.

About 1,500 eye camps are held each year, with community organizers convincing patients to come. A team from Aravind tests vision, and those needing cataract surgery receive patient counseling and are taken immediately for surgery. Those needing refraction receive their eyeglasses immediately after they receive their prescription. If the eye camp is on a Sunday, patients go to the hospital that day, have their surgery on Monday, and go home on Tuesday. This model achieves what Green called his law of propinquity: reducing the time between detection, treatment, and client satisfaction.

Green has also worked with programs in Bangladesh, China, Egypt, Guatemala, Nepal, and other countries, as well as in San Francisco. These programs perform many thousands of surgeries, many for free. For example, the Lumbini Eye Hospital in Nepal has done 47,000 surgeries, 70 percent for $33.00, 20 percent for $78.00, and 10 percent for free, while producing a profit of $220,000. "Nepal is 1 of the 10 poorest countries in the world," he observed, "and yet Nepal has found a way to serve all with eye care needs and with profit."

The cost advantage at Aravind is significantly influenced by higher labor productivity and not just lower labor costs, said Green. A cataract surgery that could cost almost $500 in a developed country can be done for just a couple of dollars in Aravind. Even if the prices from developed countries were applied to the Aravind staff, the surgery would cost only about $80.00, "which shows how there is a level of efficiency that has been achieved that the West would do well to emulate."

Green has also worked with programs to develop affordable products. For example, a company established in 1992 to make intraocular lenses now has about 10 percent of the global market, selling more than 2 million lenses per year. The Aurolab price for a lens is about $3.50, compared with more than $100.00 for its competitors. The company also makes surgical suture and pharmaceuticals for prices far below those of competitors.

By pricing its products for affordability, the company changes the competitive landscape. For example, it still has a 40 percent margin on its lenses. "It has to do with how you sculpt the business model, not only your cost but your margin," Green said. Furthermore, by providing products for much lower costs that are tuned to the needs of lower-income people, the company increases the use of those products. Cataract surgeries in India went from 800,000 to 6 million in just one decade, driven by a newly competitive ophthalmic industry. That is "something that you really don't see in the United States," said Green. "You don't really see price competition in the medical system."

Applying the Model to Hearing

Green is now applying the same model to hearing. The World Health Organization estimates that 360 million people around the world have disabling hearing loss (WHO, 2014). Yet according to Green, only about 7 million hearing aids are sold each year, and only 10 percent of those go to the developing world. These numbers have remained constant over the past decade, Green pointed out, and will remain so unless the industry experiences significant disruption with regard to pricing, distribution, and accessibility to the customer.

Green cofounded Sound World Solutions to provide amplification in real-world environments, easier access, greater availability, lower prices, and simpler processes for buying, fitting, and using the product. The technology platform that Sound World Solutions has devised is a Bluetooth-enabled hearing device that attaches to the ear. A smartphone application provides a 2-minute assessment of listening preferences and programming, and the device can be adjusted using a smartphone or the controls on the device itself. It works with iPhones or with Android-enabled phones and with Apple or PC computers. Green asserted that it has excellent directionality and noise control for both telephone and amplification mode and is the smallest Bluetooth headset in the market. It can be used both as a personal amplifier (with a limited output of 106 dB) and as a hearing aid (with a maximum output of 130 dB with 70 dB of gain). The fit is customized through an assortment of ear tips that are made out of proprietary material to reduce feedback and enable fitting for severe hearing loss without the need for a custom mold. For the behind-the-ear version, the rechargeable battery has a 16-hour life.

Green said the strategy for emerging markets is to work through preexisting programs, such as social enterprise networks, government programs, doctors' offices, and eye care programs. A training program teaches technicians how to fit the product. As a result, Green and his colleagues are able to reach beyond existing enterprises to enable entrepreneurial growth and increase access to hearing health care. In the United States, the product will be spread to underserved communities through federally qualified health care centers, American Indian clinics, Spanish-speaking clinics, county health departments, and home health care agencies. It is a business model "that makes hearing affordable and accessible to all," Green concluded.

During the discussion period, a question was raised about the FDA allowing a self-assessment test on a hearing device tied to the purchase of a hearing aid. Green noted that the test is not conducting a hearing assessment. It is intended to help a person decide on a listening preference. People have access to the controls so they can adjust the device while wearing it in different environments. When sold as a personal amplifier, the output of the device is also limited to 106 dB so that people do not damage their hearing even if they make an error in adjustments.

"We hope to shake things up," said Green. "We hope that hearing aid companies and audiology will join us in shaping different market forces that serve a much greater number of people."

INCLUSIVE DESIGN

Valerie Fletcher
Institute for Human Centered Design

The Institute for Human Centered Design is an international education and design nonprofit organization dedicated to enhancing the experiences of people of all ages and abilities through excellence in design. It is based on two core ideas, said Valerie Fletcher, the institute's executive director. First, design powerfully and profoundly influences everyone's sense of confidence, comfort, and control. Second, variation in ability is ordinary, not special, and affects most people for at least part of their lives.

Inclusive, universal, or human-centered design is a core concept of social sustainability, said Fletcher. People live longer today than they did in the past, and they have a higher standard of living. Environmental sustainability is also a growing concern and links social sustainability with respect for human diversity and interdependence, with the need for evidence, and with the long view. Inclusive design is built on a base of accessibility. This requirement intends to support equality of experience, as codified in the Rehabilitation Act of 1973, said Fletcher. Thus, whatever information is written or spoken should be as clear and understandable to people with disabilities as it is for people who do not have disabilities, Fletcher observed. But what this principle means for hearing is still in many cases a mystery.

Drivers of Inclusive Design

Global aging is the number one catalyst for inclusive design, said Fletcher (see Figure 6-1). According to Fletcher, every day 10,000 baby boomers turn 64 in the United States, and this will keep happening until 2031. "That anyone can ignore that is astonishing to me, and yet we do." Americans have what the social historian Barbara Defoe Whitehead called

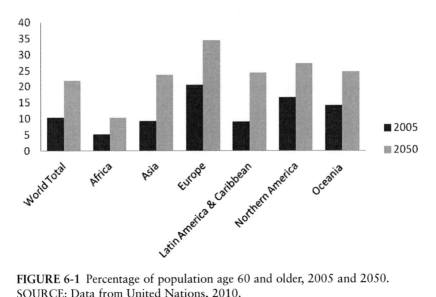

FIGURE 6-1 Percentage of population age 60 and older, 2005 and 2050.
SOURCE: Data from United Nations, 2010.

"an aging society and an adolescent culture," said Fletcher: "I sometimes feel hopeful that we are moving from that, but not very hopeful."

The second catalyst for inclusive design is disability. One in seven people on the planet has a disability, 80 percent of them in the developing world, said Fletcher. In the United States, the most common reasons for functional limitations are arthritis, back problems, heart disease, and respiratory disease. More than 55 million adults in the United States have a disability, including half of people older than age 65. Furthermore, these statistics do not count sensory or cognitive losses. "Nonapparent conditions are the norm," according to Fletcher.

Reframing the Role of Design

Inclusive design is a framework for the design of places, things, information, communication, and policy that focuses on the widest range of people operating in the widest range of situations without special or separate design provisions. As Fletcher said, the idea is human-centered design of everything with everyone in mind. According to a set of principles developed by a group of U.S. organizations in 1997, universal design calls for the following:

- Equitable use
- Flexibility in use

- Simple, intuitive use
- Perceptible information
- Tolerance for error
- Low physical effort
- Size and space for approach and use

On an international level, Fletcher said, the World Health Organization has recommended universal design as the most promising framework for identifying the facilitators that would minimize disability and support independence and full community integration. Similarly, the Madrid International Plan of Action on Aging calls for ensuring enabling and supporting environments. And the United Nations Convention on the Human Rights of People with Disabilities calls for respect, nondiscrimination, participation, inclusive design, equality, and accessibility. "We are talking about an aspiration for thriving in a world in which we cannot afford, given the volume of functional limitation, anything less," said Fletcher.

Fletcher cited several examples where inclusive design can significantly improve lives. One is to reduce the confusion felt by people taking medicines by designing better packaging and clear labeling of the medicines. "My father, who takes 11 drugs every day, does not have this," said Fletcher. "He is legally blind and struggles with 11 tubes with white caps, none of which he can read." Another example involved the redesign of a hospital in Singapore to be more patient centered. For example, in every room, at every shift, the names and photos of staff on shift are posted on the walls so that patients know who is taking care of them. Fletcher also mentioned a tablet that the Duke Cancer Center uses to screen the symptoms of patients. While in the waiting rooms, patients fill out a survey of 88 questions, rating their symptoms on a scale of 1 to 10. In this way, patients can report private matters to oncologists quickly and efficiently.

Finally, a focus on acoustics in building design, which is often neglected in design and construction because of cost considerations, can help make communication universal. For example, meeting rooms and conference tables can be engineered to help others see people speaking, recognizing the importance of visual connection to speech.

Different countries approach these issues differently, Fletcher noted. Cabs, subway stations, and museums are looped in London. The Kabukiza Kabuki Theater in Japan provides tablets with a guide for context and a script for narrative. A fire alarm company in Tokyo has even created a scented fire alarm, with tests on sleeping people showing that almost all the hearing-impaired people exposed to the odor of wasabi woke up within 2-and-a-half minutes of exposure. "You don't have to worry about whether your telecoil is turned on."

Design for people with disabilities and mainstream design can inspire, provoke, and radically change each other, Fletcher said. Hearing aids that look like jewelry and inexpensive solar-powered hearing aids are just two examples.

Inclusive design still faces an enormous research agenda, Fletcher concluded. It is an idea related to values more than evidence. But attitudes are changing, at least in some countries, she said. The Japanese, for example, are conducting research and development from the first conceptual design conversations. "They feel that they have a stake in figuring out how to maximize independence for as long as possible. They feel that they have an obligation, as a culture in an aging society, to make a difference."

During the discussion period, a workshop participant made the important point that technologies for some people with hearing loss need to be very simple. For example, older people can be very intimidated by cell phones, she said. "We have pictures of my mother's cell phone and her remote control for her TV set. This may sound surprising to you, but my mother very often mixes up the remote control for the TV set with her cell phone. This is the level we have to be thinking about. We need to be thinking about hearing devices that the older aging population can put on and use. If they can't operate it, they are not going to use it." Even with cochlear implants, people may not have the manual dexterity to operate the controls. "We are talking not about 60-year-olds who are used to using computers. We are talking about older people who very often don't have that," said this participant.

7

Contemporary Issues in Hearing Health Care

Policies and practices outside of the hearing health care system can have a substantial influence on that system. Five speakers at the workshop described the effects of three such outside influences: health goals established for the American people, changes in the health care system in general, and research being pursued by the National Institute on Deafness and Other Communication Disorders (NIDCD) of the National Institutes of Health (NIH).

HEALTHY PEOPLE 2020

Howard J. Hoffman
NIDCD/NIH

The *Healthy People* initiative was designed not as a federal initiative but as a national one with participation from nongovernmental organizations, state health agencies, professional associations, academic researchers, multiple federal agencies, and state and local stakeholders, said Howard Hoffman, director of the Epidemiology and Statistics Program at NIDCD/NIH. As Green and Fielding (2012, p. 451) observed, "The quantified objectives at the center of the initiative were a product of continuous balancing of changing science and political or social concerns and priorities along with national and state or special population needs."

In 1979 the first *Healthy People* plan was drafted on the basis of a surgeon general's report (DHEW, 1979) and an IOM report (IOM, 1978) urging a redirection of health policy toward prevention and health promotion. That plan had five objectives for the year 1990 in health promotion, five in health protection, and five in preventive health services. Since then, the number of objectives has steadily grown; the plan for 2020 includes 42 topic areas, each of which has numerous objectives.

One change for 2020 is that hearing has been separated from vision. Still, the National Health Interview Survey has been asking questions about hearing since 1990, and the number of hearing questions has expanded over that period. For example, the 2002 survey asked, "What was the MAIN cause of your hearing loss or deafness?" Responses were as follows: present at birth (3.1 percent), ear infections or other infections (8.1 percent), ear injury or surgery (3.1 percent), brief loud sound (10.3 percent), noise exposure (25.3 percent), aging (29.9 percent), some other cause (10.7 percent), and don't know cause (8.8 percent). The National Health and Nutrition Examination Survey (NHANES) has also included questions about hearing in the past, though the most recent survey focused on taste and smell rather than hearing. Together, these data sources have produced national estimates and age-specific prevalences of hearing loss, tinnitus, hearing exams, use of hearing protection, and use of hearing aids. These surveys have also produced information about comorbidities and risk factors for hearing loss.

In the area of "hearing and other sensory or communications disorders," the *Healthy People 2020* objectives include goals in not just hearing but newborn hearing screening; ear infections; tinnitus; balance and dizziness; and voice, speech, and language. For example, one goal is to "increase the proportion of persons with hearing impairments who have ever used a hearing aid or assistive listening devices or who have cochlear implants," with subgoals for particular age groups and technologies. The subgoals call for improvements of only 10 percent by 2020 over a baseline amount, noted Hoffman. "They are not meant to be unreachable targets. They are meant to be something that could be achieved." Similar goals cover hearing examinations, the use of hearing aids, cochlear implant surgeries, newborn screening, and other areas of hearing health care. Some of the goals have "taken off," Hoffman said—for example, almost all infants now receive a hearing screening during the first year of life—whereas others have met with slower change.

The *Healthy People* program is ambitious, Hoffman acknowledged. But it provides a national focus while also establishing objective and quantifiable goals that are useful at the state and local levels. The *Healthy People* tracking charts and tables provide a quick summary of progress for objectives showing improvement (or lack of improvement) over time and by key demographic groups, including race or ethnicity, education, income, gender, geography, and disability status. The data are also useful in monitoring and improving hearing outcomes for older adults, Hoffman noted. For example, tracking of hearing aid use shows gradual improvement from 2001 to 2012 for adults more than 70 years of age. "Are there strategies that can accelerate this trend?" he asked.

THE CHANGING HEALTH CARE SYSTEM

Robert Burkard
University at Buffalo

The Patient Protection and Affordable Care Act[1] (ACA) heralds major changes in the health care landscape, said Robert Burkard, professor and chair of the Department of Rehabilitation Science at the University at Buffalo. Multiple organizations have recommended moving away from a fee-for-service model and replacing it with value-based purchasing. The fee-for-service model encourages increased utilization, and more services result in more payment. "We have to get away from the assumption that more services are better outcomes," said Burkard. "We have to get into the game of how we optimize value in health care."

The biggest potential impact will be working to identify procedure groups to bundle, such as such as bundling of the current procedural terminology (CPT) codes for audiometric, acoustic immittance, and vestibular testing. With tests done together more than half the time, there is a bundle code, and physicians charge for that. They are paid less for a bundled code than for individual codes, however. The bundling of services for CPT codes probably will continue, Burkard predicted. In effect, this practice results in paying for a group of diagnostic procedures with a single payment, where the group of procedures produces both diagnostic and functional information.

Burkard also talked about the unbundling of hearing aids. Many patients ask why hearing aids are so expensive. In fact, the price usually includes many services, including taking the earmold, assessment, repair, earwax removal, counseling, and aural rehabilitation. Online and other hearing aid sales typically provide the device but not the above-listed services, making the devices substantially cheaper than when the hearing aid is bundled with services. Practices need to have a plan for how to work with patients who have purchased their hearing aids elsewhere, he said. Burkard asserted that under Medicare, if you do not charge one patient for a specific service, you cannot charge another patient for that same service. Therefore, he said, unless one unbundles, any service a practice gives away, or appears to give away, that might be billable to Medicare must be done for free for all patients. "You have to either not charge anybody," he said,

---

[1] Patient Protection and Affordable Care Act, Public Law 148, 111th Cong., 2nd sess. (March 23, 2010).

"which I don't think is saying much about the value of the service, or you have to charge everyone." Thus, he concluded, if a patient buys a hearing aid online and then asks a specialist who provides any free hearing services to hearing aid patients, that specialist might be obligated to do so.

Another aspect of the changing hearing health care landscape is the transition to ICD-10 coding. The ninth revision of the International Classification of Diseases (ICD) had about 18,000 codes, while ICD-10 has about 160,000. This provides much more specificity, but the way hearing is coded in ICD-10 "still needs work," said Burkard. ICD-10 could also be used with the International Classification of Functioning, Disability, and Health (ICF) to code levels of hearing loss severity, from zero for no problem to four for a complete problem, which provides a much broader framework to talk about the consequences of hearing loss.

The Physician Quality Reporting System was designed by CMS to improve the quality of care for Medicare beneficiaries. The ACA includes a transition from incentives for participation to penalties for nonparticipation. Still, there are currently few measures specific to audiology. The Audiology Quality Consortium, which consists of ten audiology organizations, is currently drafting measures for use—speech-in-noise testing for cochlear implant referral, functional communication ability, tinnitus screening and evaluation, ototoxic baseline measurement and monitoring, and vestibular testing—and is considering more.

The ACA describes 10 essential health benefits to be covered by health insurance exchanges and Medicaid. But the only benefits even partly related to hearing are in two categories: (1) rehabilitative and habilitative services and devices and (2) prevention and wellness services. If hearing services are not included as an essential health benefit, it seems unlikely that most accountable care organizations will include them, said Burkard. "We need to make our hearing services essential," he said. "We need evidence that what we do makes a significant difference in outcomes."

Burkard pointed out that the various professional organizations representing audiologists do not agree on the various legislative approaches for enhancing the ability of audiologists to provide optimal services. The American Academy of Audiology supports direct access, he said, whereas the American Speech-Language-Hearing Association supports comprehensive Medicare coverage of audiology services, which would allow audiologists to be reimbursed by Medicare for treatment services. The Academy of Doctors of Audiology supports limited license physician status for audiologists, direct access, and expanded audiology benefits under Medicare.

Audiologists and otolaryngologists do not always cooperate, Burkard observed. Despite evidence that audiologists are able to diagnose hearing conditions associated with significant morbidity and mortality (and thus make appropriate medical referrals), opposition is strong for direct access to audiology. The American Academy of Otolaryngology–Head and Neck Surgery strongly opposes direct access for audiology, he said. In light of this opposition, Burkard added, a bill promoting direct access for audiology (proposed by the American Academy of Audiology) is not likely to be supported. According to Burkard, "If we want to make it possible for more elders to live independently longer, to reduce medical noncompliance because those elders with hearing loss do not understand what their physician is telling them, and to improve their quality of life, we must support legislation that mandates that Medicare cover the costs of hearing aids and allow audiologists to be reimbursed for their rehabilitative services."

Interprofessional education has been a hot topic for more than a decade, Burkard observed, and speech and hearing have been a focus of attention. But there is no clear evidence that interprofessional education leads to increased value in health care, especially in hearing services, he pointed out.

At the end of his presentation, Burkard listed several priority areas that he proposed needed research. First, he argued that the audiogram is not an optimal functional measure of hearing, so research is needed for better measures, including disability scales and speech-in-noise measures. Second, he recommended a move away from a diseased-based scale of hearing loss (e.g., the ICD-10) to a functional-based scale (e.g., ICF). Third, he recommended more research on the differential diagnosis of the many causes of sensorineural hearing loss. Fourth, he suggested that while correlational research (such as between hearing loss and dementia) is important, this approach does not demonstrate cause and effect; he added that findings to date do not mean that treatment of hearing loss will reduce rates of dementia, and therefore more data are needed to support the value of adult hearing loss screening. Fifth, Burkard argued that reimbursement by Medicare is seriously flawed, and a better valuation system for CPT codes is needed. Finally, he recommended studies on the value of direct access to audiologists and what happens to quality of care when audiologists are reimbursed by Medicare to provide rehabilitative services.

NIDCD RESEARCH WORKING GROUP ON ACCESSIBLE AND AFFORDABLE HEARING HEALTH CARE

Amy M. Donahue, NIDCD/NIH
Judy R. Dubno, Medical University of South Carolina
Lucille B. Beck, U.S. Department of Veterans Affairs

In 2009 the NIDCD conducted a Research Working Group on Accessible and Affordable Hearing Healthcare for Adults with Mild to Moderate Hearing Loss. The working group looked at the hearing health care system as whole from a public health perspective and with the goal of increasing the number of individuals receiving quality hearing health care. It developed a research agenda aimed at delivering effective, affordable, and deliverable hearing health care access and outcomes to those who need them. It also wanted those outcomes to be implementable and sustainable in clinical and community settings and to complement and supplement, not replace, current paradigms. Amy Donahue, deputy director of the Division of Scientific Programs at NIDCD; Judy Dubno, professor in the Department of Otolaryngology—Head and Neck Surgery at the Medical University of South Carolina in Charleston; and Lucille Beck, chief consultant for rehabilitation and prosthetic services in the Veterans Health Administration for the Department of Veterans Affairs, described the working group's background and recommendations.

Working Group Background and Rationale

The working group focused on adults of all ages with mild to moderate hearing loss, not just older Americans. But mild to moderate hearing loss represents the hearing status of many older Americans, and they are least likely to have had a hearing screening assessment or use a hearing aid for one of many reasons. Yet early intervention may lead to better outcomes, Donahue noted. In addition, many of these individuals are still active in the workforce, and many will transition to severe hearing loss and need more complex interventions and services in later years.

Access is as important as affordability, she said. Today, there are no readily accessible, low-cost ways for U.S. adults to get their hearing screened. Instead, there are multiple entry points marked by competing interests, including family practitioners, audiologists, hearing aid specialists, and otolaryngologists. Also, obtaining a device through traditional delivery models is a multi-visit process, requiring a visit to a physician and a specialist in audiology. Direct-to-consumer marketing heretofore has been the primary source of low-cost hearing aids, available through the Internet, magazines, newspapers, but "consumer beware," said Donahue. "We need better alternatives."

According to Donahue, the average out-of-pocket cost of one hearing aid, including devices and services, is approximately $1,800. About 70 percent of people require two aids. The life span of hearing aids is approximately 4 to 6 years, after which replacement costs repeat the expense. Yet 35 percent of American households have an income of less than $35,000 per year, and the median household income in America is $50,000 per year. Different segments of the population likely have different price points, and there are limited scientific data on the specific impact of costs on adoption rates. But among nonadopters, cost is cited as the primary reason for not getting a hearing aid. Two-thirds of these people said that they would get a hearing aid if insurance or other programs provided 100 percent coverage, and 47 percent said they were likely to get a hearing aid if the price did not exceed $500. "Beyond the purchase of a home or a car, hearing aids and services can be the third most expensive purchase for many Americans with hearing loss over time." But hearing health care is not covered by Medicare or most insurance plans. Instead, people rely on Lions Clubs, loaner banks, and philanthropic organizations, which "is not an acceptable public health solution."

One of NIH's missions is to close gaps in health disparities, including those among racial and ethnic minorities, the urban and rural poor, and the medically underserved. Acquiring hearing health care may be especially challenging for the working poor. "It is important that we remain conscious of the underserved and the economically less advantaged," said Donahue.

Donahue elaborated on rapid changes in new and emerging technologies (e.g., automated assessment and hearing aid fitting, smartphone capabilities) as well as changing service delivery paradigms that offer potential for making hearing health care more accessible and affordable. She also provided information on the professional tensions among hearing health care providers and their lack of agreement on legislative strategies to address hearing health care.

Prioritized Recommendations of the NIDCD Research Working Group

The research recommendations focused on current and evolving technologies and strategies that are effective, accessible, and affordable; that reflect the demographics and socioeconomic capacities of the U.S. population; and that are practical and feasible for the near future. The members of the working group selected their highest-priority recommendations from a list of more than 70 recommendations. These were organized into 10 different areas:

- Access
- Screening
- Assessment
- Hearing aid technologies
- Patient variables
- Aftercare needs
- Delivery systems
- Workforce and training of hearing health care professionals
- Medical evaluation and regulatory issues
- Overarching topics

Donahue did not go through all the recommendations at the workshop, but she provided an overview of several of the most important. First, an overarching research recommendation of the working group is to understand the benefits of hearing health care for general health, economic health, lifestyle, well-being, and family life. In the area of access, a better understanding is needed of such variables as complexity of services, costs, insurance and subsidies, location, and referral networks, she said. At the same time, patient-centered variables need to be studied, including needs and concerns, values, socioeconomic status, attitudes, stigma, and culture.

Barriers to hearing screening need to be evaluated, said Donahue, including availability, cost, insurance coverage, referral patterns, and the effect of health care settings. The best screening methods need to be determined in terms of sensitivity, specificity, follow-up rates, and long-term benefits to hearing health. Accessible screening paradigms are needed for emerging technologies and target populations.

In the area of assessment, the quality and accuracy of audiometry needs to be determined in different health care settings using different means of delivery, Donahue continued. The necessary components of assessment batteries, including cognitive and psychosocial components, need to be determined to guide the fitting of hearing aids and other interventions.

Hearing aid technology variables that predict success and influence market penetration rates need to be identified, Donahue said, including the minimal level of technology needed to achieve success. The effectiveness of various technologies for various populations also needs to be determined. Patient variables that predict success and influence market penetration rates (such as motivation, perceived need, age, socioeconomic status, and culture) also need to be identified, she said.

A standard set of measures to determine the success of hearing health care and better determination of how and when to measure outcomes would benefit the field, she added. For aftercare needs, the information and patient education needed for various service delivery models should be explored, she said.

Innovative delivery systems, such as mHealth, could be used for hearing health care. There is a need to modify current models, both the system and the provider, to increase access and affordability. With such changes, the necessary knowledge, skills, and abilities of hearing health care providers should be determined, whether in a traditional or nontraditional setting.

Finally, under medical evaluation and regulatory issues, Donahue asked whether the FDA regulations provide protection for patients or whether they create a barrier for access, thereby delaying necessary intervention. Needed evidence includes the appropriate medical evaluation for using a hearing aid, the percentage opting for a medical waiver, the prevalence of treatable causes of hearing loss in adults seeking hearing aids, and the ability of consumers to detect treatable hearing loss.

NIDCD widely distributed and discussed the working group's report.[2] It has also encouraged grant applications through both traditional and unique NIH funding mechanisms. Box 7-1 lists some of the grants active at the time of the IOM-NRC workshop.

CHALLENGES AND OPPORTUNITIES

Finally, Donahue listed some of the challenges and opportunities in hearing health care. The pool of clinician-researchers in audiology and otolaryngology is small, she said. Interest in hearing loss research among other relevant professions—including gerontology, primary care, family medicine, outcomes, health services, public health, and epidemiology—is limited. Finally, research conducted in communities in partnership with researchers, outside an academic medical center, has been limited.

"This [IOM-NRC] workshop is a real opportunity to encourage engagement of the larger research community in this endeavor," said Donahue. "These research recommendations remain timely and important." NIDCD has been able to maintain hearing health care as a priority research area despite tight funding, and support from NIDCD leadership, staff, and the institute's advisory council remains strong. Funding applications grew from 4 in fiscal year 2011 and less than $1 million to 15 in fiscal year 2013 and more than $4 million. Finally, the Senate report language for the institute's fiscal year 2013 appropriations says, "The Committee strongly urges NIDCD to support research grants that could lead to less expensive hearing aids, so such aids could become accessible and affordable to more people."

During the discussion period, Margaret Wallhagen emphasized the difficulty of conducting community-based research and partnerships. Trying to conduct research in a clinical setting requires overcoming major barriers, such as time, privacy, and ongoing changes in the health care system. Yet these studies are essential to figure out what will work in a real-world setting. In response, Donahue pointed to innovative practice-based networks where a group of practitioners come together and agree to participate in research. They use streamlined processes for recruitment and institutional review board approvals while drawing on their own patient populations to contribute to the overall project. For example, the Creating Healthcare Excellence through Education and Research project at the Duke Clinical Research Institute is a practice-based network involving otolaryngology, audiology, and speech pathology. Another example cited was the Great

---

[2] The report is available at http://www.nidcd.nih.gov/funding/programs/09HHC/Pages/summary.aspx (accessed February 28, 2014).

BOX 7-1
Research Projects on Hearing Health Care Being Funded by
NIDCD at the Time of the Workshop

Effectiveness of Basic and Premium Hearing Aid Features for Older Adults: Comparing the effectiveness of basic-level and premium-level hearing aids

Minimal Technologies for Hearing Aid Success in Older Adults: Relationship between technology level and real-world effectiveness using wireless smartphones as part of outcome measurement system

Efficacy of a Low-Cost Hearing Aid and Comparison of Service Delivery Models: Clinical trial including service-delivery model (current best practices and over-the-counter simulation) and purchase price (low and typical)

Ability of Consumers and Audiologists to Detect Ear Disease Prior to Hearing Aid Use: Evidence relevant to the FDA-required medical evaluation with waiver option

Reduction of Disparities in Access to Hearing Health Care on the U.S.-Mexico Border: Testing the effectiveness of an innovative community health worker intervention (Promotora), used for other chronic conditions, to expand hearing health care access among older adults facing health disparities

User-Centered Control of Hearing Aid Signal Processing—Allows users to select their desired signal processing parameter values on mobile devices that communicate wirelessly with hearing aids

Improvement of Amplification Outcomes in Noise by Self-Directed Hearing Aid Fitting: Self-fitting with wireless control of hearing aids to explore preferred settings in noise—allow users to custom fit algorithms for greater success in background noise in daily use

Primary Care Intervention Promoting Hearing Health Care Service Access and Use: Within a primary care setting, testing the effectiveness of three protocols on subsequent access to and use of hearing health care services

Community-Based Kiosks for Hearing Screening and Education: Within four community-based centers, testing the effectiveness of five hearing screening paradigms for hearing health care follow-up and hearing aid uptake

A National Screening Test for Hearing, Administered by Telephone: A U.S. version of a telephone-administered screening test that has been implemented in Australia, France, Germany, the Netherlands, and the United Kingdom

Wireless and Noise Attenuating Headset for Automatic Hearing Screening: Development of a mobile platform hearing screening device designed for use at point-of-care locations with limited personnel resources

Lakes Practice into Research Network, a primary care research network in Michigan.

Lucille Beck, who is the chief consultant for rehabilitation and prosthetics, as well as the chief of the audiology and speech language pathology services at the U.S. Department of Veterans Affairs, also pointed to funding through the VA for the Health Services Research Community, which looks at the context of service delivery in the real world. This interdisciplinary research is looking at cross-disciplinary teams of physicians, nurses, social workers, and community service workers all working on behalf of patients.

8

Collaborative Strategies for the Future

A wide range of organizations are involved with issues related to hearing loss, many of which were represented at the workshop. In the workshop's final session, representatives of three of these organizations described some of the ways in which they are working on hearing loss, providing examples of ways in which organizations can produce progress on the issue. Workshop participants then closed the workshop by offering their perspectives on the 2 days of deliberations.

THE AMERICAN PUBLIC HEALTH ASSOCIATION

Regina Davis Moss
American Public Health Association

The public health implications of age-related hearing loss go far beyond the immediate threat to the individual, said Regina Davis Moss, associate executive director of public health policy and practice for the American Public Health Association (APHA). Age-related hearing loss has been linked to social isolation, depression, and anxiety, which can lead to other public health and safety issues. Yet many people seek treatment too late in the United States and worldwide.

Public health is a community-based approach that makes use of various settings for reaching different populations. These settings include not just physicians' offices, hospitals, and nursing facilities but also places of worship, community-based programs, and retirement communities, among others.

The APHA has issued several policy statements related to hearing. It advocates for early and cost-effective screening programs for at-risk populations, followed by careful evaluation and treatment. It also supports public education about conditions, warning signs, and the importance of seeking treatment. This public education includes preventive measures, such as hearing protection among younger people, said Moss. In addition, the APHA promotes a research agenda that includes such issues as screening for asymptomatic individuals.

THE AMERICAN GERIATRICS SOCIETY

James Pacala
University of Minnesota Medical School

Although representing the American Geriatrics Society (AGS) at the workshop, James Pacala, distinguished teaching professor at the University of Minnesota Medical School, offered his personal impressions of the issues surrounding hearing loss. He works in an underserved community in South Minneapolis at a busy clinic that trains residents, mental health workers, and pharmacists. The average age of his patients is about 85, and over the course of the day he is likely to use three different interpreters. "It is a challenging setting to deliver care."

Pacala identified six hurdles to providing good hearing health care. First, everything in medicine is predicated on patient visits, he said, but most of the things that happen to patients occur outside visits. Second, the demand for evidence ignores the fact that many things done in medicine do not have a solid evidence base but are still important. Third, he described "the tyranny of the acute" in which the physician focuses attention on a patient's immediate problems and tends to overlook longer-term issues such as hearing loss. Fourth, addressing chronic diseases such as diabetes can consume all of the time available for physician-delivered care. Fifth, shifting focus to prevention and health maintenance adds to the number of things that need to be covered in a family medicine practice. And, sixth, many important health problems are neglected in medical education and training, and hearing is one.

Acting alone, physicians cannot overcome these hurdles, he said; instead, health policies need to change to remove the barriers to better hearing health care. For example, structural and financial barriers around the way care is provided and organized can stymie hearing health care. Innovations such as patient-centered medical homes and accountable care organizations are moving in a positive direction, said Pacala, but "we have a long way to go." Also, in the area of policy, the financial burdens of assisted listening devices and hearing aids need to be reduced, he said.

Awareness is another important issue. "We need to continue to pound the pavement and increase awareness about this problem," he said. For example, the AGS, through its Health in Aging Foundation, provides an Aging and Health A to Z webpage through which patients can access information on hearing loss and related issues.[1]

Finally, much more research is needed on how to partner medicine, public health, and technology to come together to create better environments and better ways of solving the problem, Pacala said. Research into implementation is also critical to figure out how best to provide help for older adults.

AARP

Charlotte Yeh
AARP

Charlotte Yeh, chief medical officer for AARP Services, Inc., began her presentation by noting that her life's experiences added to her thoughts about hearing loss: her role at AARP Services is to improve the experience of care for individuals over the age of 50, her experience as an emergency medicine physician reinforced the importance of communication, and her father's experience with progressive hearing loss gave her personal insights. (See Box 8-1.)

BOX 8-1
The Difference That Hearing Can Make

Throughout the workshop, presenters and other participants offered accounts of the effects that hearing loss has had on their lives and on the lives of their family members. The story told by Charlotte Yeh, chief medical officer for AARP Services, Inc., was a good example: "My father spent 15 years with progressive hearing loss. . . . Finally, he got his hearing aid, and all of a sudden he wasn't shuffling. He was walking with confidence. All of a sudden he wasn't bent over. He was animated; he was telling jokes. He wasn't sitting quietly in the corner; he was part of the family. He was telling jokes, laughing, enjoying his children and grandchildren in a way I haven't seen since I was a child. As you can tell, I have a lot of personal thoughts and passion about this vision of what we can do with hearing and hearing loss."

---

[1] See http://www.healthinaging.org/aging-and-health-a-to-z (accessed March 31, 2014).

The major message delivered by Yeh is that consumer engagement is the key to changing the conversation. The rest of health care is already pursing such aspects of consumer engagement as behavior change and motivation. Those involved with hearing issues need to do the same thing, said Yeh, and this effort needs to encompass not just consumers but industry, researchers, and other stakeholders.

According to Yeh, changing the conversation has three components. First, the conversation needs to be about the heart and mind of the consumer. Consumer retail does this well, she observed. It does not focus on loss but what is to be gained. Similarly, conversations about hearing loss could focus on the gain from social interactions, family connections, and workplace productivity. Hearing loss "is not a standalone disability. It is integral to everything we do every single day." According to a study of adults with a Medicare Supplement plan (Hawkins et al., 2012), hearing loss has a greater impact on quality of life than diabetes, heart disease, coronary artery disease, hypertension, or any other medical condition, Yeh reported. Similarly, a survey conducted in 2011 of people older than 50 found that 85 percent said that hearing is very important to their quality of life, 76 percent said it is personally important to their lives, and 68 percent said that not enough attention is paid to hearing loss as an important health care concern (AARP/ASHA, 2011). Yet conversations about medical issues tend to revolve around conditions other than hearing. "More people have had colonoscopies than hearing tests," said Yeh. "What is wrong with this prevention message, if you think about it?"

The same survey (AARP/ASHA, 2011) also asked about issues of stigma, and Yeh said it is time to "blow away that myth." In fact, 64 percent of respondents said that they did not think that having hearing aids meant a person was getting old. Two-thirds said that having a hearing aid did not matter to others, and 71 percent said they would not worry if other people saw them with the hearing aid. "The paradigms are shifting," said Yeh.

About two-thirds also said that they would get a hearing test if their hearing were hurting their relationships with their family, and 59 percent said they would be tested if their hearing was becoming a burden on the family. According to AARP research, said Yeh, the top things on people's minds are their relationship with others, whether they are a burden on their family, and their mental alertness. Emphasizing the importance of good hearing is not a negative thing, said Yeh. It offers the promise of a good life.

Yeh also pointed out that the conversation about hearing needs to reflect the fact that hearing needs range along a continuum, as does acceptance of the issue. The conversation should be about "where you are on the stage of acceptance, what are the products and capabilities, and how do we help people adjust and move through that continuum," she said. This facet of the conversation also entails behavior change, motivation, patient activation, and readiness to change. "Those are things that we are talking about in health care. We should be talking about them in hearing loss as well."

Finally, Yeh discussed the issue of affordability, including costs, coverage, reimbursement, and "respect for the time and convenience of the consumer." Industry needs to continue to work on how to make the technology easier to use, better in noisy situations, and less costly, she said.

Baby boomers are used to getting things done, she concluded. "We are the ones who brought civil rights. We put a man on the moon. We had rock and roll, which is why we have hearing loss, and we brought Woodstock. If this isn't a generation that can bring about that change, I don't know what else is."

PARTICIPANTS' REFLECTIONS ON THE WORKSHOP

At the end of the workshop, speakers and participants were asked to provide their reflections on the 2 days of presentations and discussions. James Firman, National Council on Aging, began by calling attention to the need to tie hearing to quality-of-life issues. Policy makers are concerned that people be able to continue to contribute to society, whether through work, volunteer activities, or involvement with their families and communities. Good hearing is essential to that connection, said Firman.

He also pointed out that so many older adults have hearing loss that the only way to address the problem comprehensively is through universal design. Loops and other devices to improve hearing need to be the rule rather than the exception, he said, just as closed captioning on television has become common.

Wen Chen, National Institute on Aging, emphasized the importance of communicating about age-related hearing loss to the older adult community in general. Many options are available for older adults with hearing loss, but some of those options are bound to be confusing, especially in areas where technology is advancing rapidly. Perhaps an emphasis on the outcomes of technology—such as hearing better in noise—would be a more powerful message than one that centers on the technologies themselves, such as telecoils and loops.

James Appleby, Gerontological Society of America, recommended that more research be conducted to demonstrate that hearing interventions have value not only in improving health and economic outcomes but also in redirecting the trajectories of people's lives. Such outcomes can help make the case for greater investment in hearing interventions. He also recommended that more attention be given to the issue of reducing stigma by reframing the issue of hearing loss around engagement and the need for action.

Anna Gilmore Hall, Hearing Loss Association of America, urged changing the conversation to focus on ways of living successfully with hearing loss. There are many different ways to live successfully with hearing loss, she noted, especially given the many new technologies that are becoming available.

Robert Burkard, University at Buffalo, said that hearing health care should become an essential health benefit within the broader context of health care reform. Burkard also urged the FDA to push harder on enforcing honesty in advertisements about hearing technologies.

Composer Richard Einhorn emphasized the need for hearing health care and hearing devices to be affordable, adding that addressing the issue requires fundamental changes in the FDA regulations. Although many players are involved in regulations, he added, change is possible that would benefit all stakeholders, including consumers and companies. He also wondered why age-related hearing loss is not higher on the agenda of gerontology, public health, and other health disciplines. One beneficial product of the workshop could be raising the profile of the issue, he said.

Barbara E. Weinstein, Graduate School and University Center of the City University of New York, recommended that the hearing health care delivery system be reframed to put the patient at the center of the audiological assessment. People come to audiologists because they have difficulties in certain areas, and they need to leave audiologists' offices with solutions. Someone may not be ready for a $6,000 hearing aid; they may only have problems with the television. That person may need just an infrared system for the television or one of the many varieties of personal amplifiers that are inexpensive and may increase the loudness enough to contribute to the enjoyment of television viewing. Both policies and medical practices should encourage those kinds of solutions, Weinstein said.

Author Katherine Bouton pointed to the need to get the entire population involved in the conversation, not just those with hearing loss. "They need to understand that this is, if not a universal problem, close to it." Part of the solution will be making hearing aids as affordable, ubiquitous, and effective as glasses. People today often see hearing loss as a sign of aging and view correction as complicated and ineffective, so they keep their difficulties to themselves, she said.

Valerie Fletcher, Institute for Human Centered Design, thought that many vignettes could be compiled of successful efforts to counter hearing loss involving collaborative efforts among clinicians, patients, and technologists. Such a compilation "would go a long way toward eradicating the assumption that nothing works very well."

Steven Barnett, University of Rochester, called for research on the conditions associated with hearing loss. His patients are concerned about what other consequences hearing loss might have, yet he has little information for them today. In addition, much more needs to be learned about the condition through more detailed questions on surveys and through increased surveillance, he said.

Sergio Guerreiro, University of Miami School of Medicine, and Alicia Spoor, Academy of Doctors of Audiology, both said that hearing health care should be a standard part of care for everyone. Hearing tests should be routinely given to patients, Guerreiro said, just as other tests are given. Physicians should ask their patients about hearing in the same way they ask about smoking, added Spoor.

Chris Roberts, Cochlear Limited, discussed the possibility of creating a disconnect between chronological aging and biological aging. With regard to hearing, reduced exposure to noise can prevent hearing losses, and audiological training can reduce loss of function. "There is a lot more that could [be done] to affect the biology of what is happening."

Brenda Battat, retired executive director of the Hearing Loss Association of America, pointed out that baby boomers express a desire to stay in their homes as they get older, but they will not be able to do so unless they address hearing problems. Hearing health care thus can have benefits for older individuals, families, and health care costs. She also agreed that the FDA regulations are out of date and that hearing aid manufacturers need to produce devices that allow individuals to hear better in noise.

Paul Mick, University of British Columbia, wanted more evidence of not just associations but also causal links between hearing loss and the physical and psychosocial effects associated with hearing loss. Such evidence would enable physicians to provide better advice for their patients and would be a force for greater funding and services. Outcomes data on interventions could have the same effect, he said. And identification of at-risk populations would help focus attention on these groups.

Finally, planning committee cochair Frank Lin noted that many organizations and perspectives were represented at the workshop, yet everyone there was focused on the issue of how to improve hearing health care for older adults. "The conversation has begun," he said.

References

AARP/ASHA (American Speech-Language-Hearing Association). 2011. *AARP/American Speech-Language-Hearing Association (ASHA) national poll on hearing health: Results summary.* http://www.asha.org/uploadedFiles/AARP-ASHA-National-Hearing-Health-Poll.pdf (accessed March 18, 2014).

Cacioppo, J. T., L. C. Hawkley, G. J. Norman, and G. G. Berntson. 2011. Social isolation. *Annals of the New York Academy of Sciences* 1231:17–22.

CEN (European Committee for Standardization). 2010. *EN 15927: Services offered by hearing aid professionals.* http://media.wix.com/ugd/c2e099_b8d0227c3d2c4664933f2 eafcc5f5bc0.pdf (accessed March 10, 2014).

Chen, D. S., J. Betz, K. Yaffe, H. N. Ayonayon, S. Kritchevsky, K. R. Martin, T. B. Harris, E. Purchase-Helzner, S. Satterfield, Q. Xue, S. Pratt, E. M. Simonsick, and F. R. Lin. In review. Association of hearing impairment with declines in physical functioning and the risk of disability in older adults.

Chia, E. M., J. J. Wang, E. Rochtchina, R. R. Cumming, P. Newall, and P. Mitchell. 2007. Hearing impairment and health-related quality of life: The Blue Mountains Hearing Study. *Ear and Hearing* 28(2):187–195.

Chien, W., and F. R. Lin. 2012. Prevalence of hearing aid use among older adults in the United States. *Archives of Internal Medicine* 172(3):292–293.

Chisolm, T., and M. Arnold. 2012. Evidence about the effectiveness of aural rehabilitation programs for adults. In *Evidence-based practice in audiology*, edited by L. Wong and L. Hickson. San Diego: Plural Publishing.

Chou, R., T. Dana, C. Bougatsos, C. Fleming, and T. Beil. 2011. *Screening for hearing loss in adults ages 50 years and older: A review of the evidence for the U.S. Preventive Services Task Force.* Evidence Synthesis No. 83, AHRQ Publication No. 11-05153-EF-1. Rockville, MD: Agency for Healthcare Research and Quality.

CMS (Centers for Medicare & Medicaid Services). 2014. *Your Medicare coverage: Hearing and balance exams & hearing aids.* http://www.medicare.gov/coverage/hearing-and-balance-exam-and-hearing-aids.html (accessed April 17, 2014).

Dalton, D. S., K. J. Cruickshanks, B. E. Klein, R. Klein, T. L. Wiley, and D. M. Nondahl. 2003. The impact of hearing loss on quality of life in older adults. *Gerontologist* 43(5):661–668.

Davis, A., P. Smith, M. Ferguson, D. Stephens, and I. Gianopoulos. 2007. Acceptability, benefits, and costs of early screening for hearing disability: A study of potential screening tests and models. *Health Technology Assessment* 11(42):1–294.

DHEW (Department of Health, Education, and Welfare). 1979. *Healthy People: The surgeon general's report on health promotion and disease prevention.* Washington, DC: U.S. Department of Health, Education, and Welfare.

Dillon, H., A. James, and J. Ginis. 1997. The Client Oriented Scale of Improvement (COSI) and its relationship to several other measures of benefit and satisfaction provided by hearing aids. *Journal of the American Academy of Audiology* 8(27):27–43.

Ferrucci, L., and S. Studenski. 2011. Clinical problems of aging. In *Harrison's Principles of Internal Medicine*, edited by D. L. Longo, A. Fauci, D. Kasper, S. Hauser, J. L. Jameson, and J. Loscalzo. New York: McGraw-Hill.

Gallacher, J., V. Ilubaera, Y. Ben-Shlomo, A. Bayer, M. Fish, W. Babisch, and P. Elwood. 2012. Auditory threshold, phonologic demand, and incident dementia. *Neurology* 79(15):1583–1590.

Genther, D. J., K. D. Frick, D. Chen, J. Betz, and F. R. Lin. 2013. Association of hearing loss with hospitalization and burden of disease in older adults. *Journal of the American Medical Association* 309(22):2322–2324.

Gilhotra, J. S., P. Mitchell, R. Ivers, and R. G. Cumming. 2001. Impaired vision and other factors associated with driving cessation in the elderly: The Blue Mountains Eye Study. *Clinical and Experimental Ophthalmology* 29(3):104–107.

Gopinath, B., L. Hickson, J. Schneider, C. M. McMahon, G. Burlutsky, S. R. Leeder, and P. Mitchell. 2012. Hearing-impaired adults are at increased risk of experiencing emotional distress and social engagement restrictions five years later. *Age and Ageing* 41(5):618–623.

Green, L. W., and J. Fielding J. 2011. The U.S. Healthy People Initiative: Its genesis and its sustainability. *Annual Review of Public Health* 32:451–470.

Hawkins, K., F. G. Bottone, Jr., R. J. Ozminkowski, S. Musich, M. Bai, R. J. Migliori, and C. S. Yeh. 2012. The prevalence of hearing impairment and its burden on the quality of life among adults with Medicare Supplement Insurance. *Quality of Life Research* 21:1135–1147.

Hawthorne, G. 2008. Perceived social isolation in a community sample: Its prevalence and correlates with aspects of peoples' lives. *Social Psychiatry and Psychiatric Epidemiology* 43(2):140–150.

Henshaw, H., and M. A. Ferguson. 2013. Efficacy of individual computer-based auditory training for people with hearing loss: A systematic review of the evidence. *PLoS ONE* 8(5):e62836.

Hickson, L., J. Wood, A. Chaparro, P. Lacherez, and R. Marszalek. 2010. Hearing impairment affects older people's ability to drive in the presence of distracters. *Journal of the American Geriatrics Society* 58(6):1097–1103.

Hogan, A., K. O'Loughlin, P. Miller, and H. Kendig. 2009. The health impact of a hearing disability on older people in Australia. *Journal of Aging and Health* 21(8):1098–1111.

Ingram, M., R. Piper, S. Kunz, C. Navarro, A. Sander, and S. Gastelum. 2012. Salud Sí: A case study for the use of participatory evaluation in creating effective and sustainable community-based health promotion. *Journal of Family and Community Health* 35(2):130–138.

IOM (Institute of Medicine). 1978. *Perspectives on health promotion and disease prevention in the United States.* Washington, DC: National Academy Press.

Johnson, D., P. Saavedra, E. Sun, A. Stageman, D. Grovet, C. Alfero, B. Skipper, W. Powell, and A. Kaufman. 2012. Community health workers and Medicaid managed care in New Mexico. *Journal of Community Health* 37(3):563–571.

Karpa, M. J., B. Gopinath, K. Beath, E. Rochtchina, R. G. Cumming, J. J. Wang, and P. Mitchell. 2010. Associations between hearing impairment and mortality risk in older persons: The Blue Mountains Hearing Study. *Annals of Epidemiology* 20(6):452–459.

Klop, W. M. C., J. J. Briaire, A. M. Stiggelbout, and J. H. M. Frijns. 2007. Cochlear implant outcomes and quality of life in adults with prelingual deafness. *Laryngoscope* 117(11):1982–1987.

Lin, F. R. 2012. Hearing loss in older adults: Who's listening? *Journal of the American Medical Association* 307(11):1147–1148.

Lin, F. R., J. K. Niparko, and L. Ferrucci. 2011a. Hearing loss prevalence in the United States. *JAMA Internal Medicine* 171(20):1851–1852.

Lin, F. R., E. J. Metter, R. J. O'Brien, S. M. Resnick, A. B. Zonderman, and L. Ferrucci. 2011b. Hearing loss and incident dementia. *Archives of Neurology* 68(2):214–220.

Lin, F. R., K. Yaffe, J. Xia, Q. L. Xue, T. B. Harris, E. Purchase-Helzner, S. Satterfield, H. N. Ayonayon, L. Ferrucci, E. M. Simonsick, and the Health ABC Study Group. 2013. Hearing loss and cognitive decline in older adults. *JAMA Internal Medicine* 173(4):293–299.

MacDonald, M. 2011. *The association between degree of hearing loss and depression in older adults*. Master's thesis. University of British Columbia, Vancouver.

Meyer, C., L. Hickson, A. Khan, D. Hartley, H. Dillon, and J. Seymour. 2011. Investigation of the actions taken by adults who failed a telephone-based hearing screen. *Ear and Hearing* 32(6):720–731.

Mulrow, C. D., C. Aguilar, J. E. Endicott, R. Velez, M. R. Tuley, W. S. Charlip, and J. A. Hill. 1990. Association between hearing impairment and the quality of life of elderly individuals. *Journal of the American Geriatrics Society* 38(1):45–50.

Peelle, J. E., V. Troiani, M. Grossman, and A. Wingfield. 2011. Hearing loss in older adults affects neural systems supporting speech comprehension. *Journal of Neuroscience* 31(35): 12638–12643.

Picard, M., S. A. Girard, M. Courteau, T. Leroux, R. Larocque, F. Turcotte, M. Lavoie, and M. Simard. 2008. Could driving safety be compromised by noise exposure at work and noise-induced hearing loss? *Traffic Injury Prevention* 9(5):489–499.

Pichora-Fuller, M. K., B. A. Schneider, and M. Daneman. 1995. How young and old adults listen to and remember speech in noise. *Journal of the Acoustical Society of America* 97(1):593–608.

Reinschmidt, K., and J. Chong. 2008. SONRISA: A curriculum toolbox for *promotores* to address mental health and diabetes. *Preventing Chronic Disease* 4(4) [serial online]. http://www.cdc.gov/pcd/issues/2007/oct/07_0021.htm (accessed March 18, 2014).

Rosenthal, E. L., J. N. Brownstein, C. H. Rush, G. R. Hirsch, A. M. Willaert, J. R. Scott, L. R. Holderby, and D. J. Fox. 2010. Community Health Workers: Part of the solution. *Health Affairs* 29(7):1338–1342.

Sabo, S., M. Ingram, K. Reinschmidt, K. Schachter, L. Jacobs, J. G. Zapien, and S. Carvajal. 2013. Predictors and a framework for fostering community advocacy as a community health worker (CHW) core function to eliminate health disparities. *American Journal of Public Health* 103(7):367–373.

Saito, H., Y. Nishiwaki, T. Michikawa, Y. Kikuchi, K. Mizutari, T. Takebayashi, and K. Ogawa. 2010. Hearing handicap predicts the development of depressive symptoms after 3 years in older community-dwelling Japanese. *Journal of the American Geriatrics Society* 58(1):93–97.

Schneider, J., B. Gopinath, M. J. Karpa, C. M. McMahon, E. Rochtchina, S. R. Leeder, and
     P. Mitchell. 2010. Hearing loss impacts on the use of community and informal supports.
     Age and Ageing 39(4):458–464.
Staten, L. K., C. Cutshaw, C. Davidson, K. Reinschmidt, R. Stewart, and D. Roe. 2012. Ef-
     fectiveness of the Pasos Adelante chronic disease prevention and control program in a
     US-Mexico border community, 2005–2008. *Preventing Chronic Disease* 9 [serial online].
     http://www.cdc.gov/pcd/issues/2012/10_0301.htm (accessed March 18, 2014).
Thorén, E., M. Svensson, A. Törnqvist, G. Andersson, P. Carlbring, and T. Lunner. 2011. Re-
     habilitative online education versus internet discussion group for hearing aid users: a ran-
     domized controlled trial. *Journal of the American Academy of Audiology* 22(5):274–285.
Uhlmann, R. F., E. B. Larson, T. S. Rees, T. D. Koepsell, and L. G. Duckert. 1989. Relationship
     of hearing impairment to dementia and cognitive dysfunction in older adults. *Journal of
     the American Medical Association* 261(13):1916–1919.
United Nations, Department of Economic and Social Affairs, Population Division. 2010.
     World population prospects: The 2006 revision, highlights. New York: United Nations.
USPSTF (U.S. Preventive Services Task Force). 2012. *Screening for hearing loss in older
     adults: U.S. Preventive Services Task Force Recommendation Statement.* http://www.
     uspreventiveservicestaskforce.org/uspstf11/adulthearing/adulthearrs.htm (accessed
     March 18, 2014).
Valente, M., H. Abrams, D. Benson, T. Chisolm, D. Citron, D. Hampton, A. Loavenbruck, T.
     Ricketts, H. Solodar, and R. Sweetow. 2006. Guidelines for the audiological management
     of adult hearing impairment. *Audiology Today* 18(5):32–35.
Ventry, I. M., and B. E. Weinstein. 1982. The hearing handicap inventory for the elderly: A
     new tool. *Ear and Hearing* 3(3):128–134.
Viljanen, A., J. Kaprio, I. Pyykkö, M. Sorri, M. Koskenvuo, and T. Rantanen. 2009. Hearing
     acuity as a predictor of walking difficulties in older women. *Journal of the American
     Geriatrics Society* 57(12):2282–2286.
Viswanathan, M., J. Kraschnewski, B. Nishikawa, L. C. Morgan, P. Thieda, A. Honeycutt,
     K. N. Lohr, and D. Jonas. 2009. *Outcomes of community health worker interventions:
     Evidence report/technology assessment no. 181.* Prepared by the RTI International–
     University of North Carolina Evidence-Based Practice Center under Contract No. 290
     2007 10056 I. AHRQ Publication No. 09-E014. Rockville, MD: Agency for Healthcare
     Research and Quality.
Wallhagen, M. I., and E. Pettengill. 2008. Hearing impairment: Significant but underassessed
     in primary care settings. *Journal of Gerontological Nursing* 34(2):36–42.
Wallhagen, M. I., W. J. Strawbridge, S. J. Shema, J. Kurata, and G. A. Kaplan. 2001. Com-
     parative impact of hearing and vision impairment on subsequent functioning. *Journal of
     the American Geriatrics Society* 49(8):1086–1092.
Weinstein, B. E., and I. M. Ventry. 1982. Hearing impairment and social isolation in the el-
     derly. *Journal of Speech, Language, and Hearing Research* 25(4):593–599.
WHO (World Health Organization). 2014. *Deafness and hearing loss: Fact sheet no. 300.*
     http://www.who.int/mediacentre/factsheets/fs300/en (accessed February 28, 2014).
Yueh, B., M. P. Collins, P. E. Souza, E. J. Boyko, C. F. Loovis, P. J. Heagerty, C. F. Liu, and
     S. C. Hedrick. 2010. Long-term effectiveness of screening for hearing loss: The screening
     for auditory impairment—which hearing assessment test (SAI-WHAT) randomized trial.
     Journal of the American Geriatrics Society 58(3):427–434.

Appendix A

Workshop Agenda

Hearing Loss and Healthy Aging: A Workshop

January 13–14, 2014

The Keck Center of the National Academies
500 Fifth Street, NW
Washington, DC 20001

Sponsored by:
IOM-NRC Forum on Aging, Disability, and Independence
Academy of Doctors of Audiology
American Academy of Audiology
American Academy of Otolaryngology–Head and Neck Surgery
American Speech-Language-Hearing Association
Cochlear Americas
European Hearing Instrument Manufacturers Association
Hearing Industries Association
Hearing Loss Association of America
Hi HealthInnovations
MED-EL Corporation, USA
National Institute on Aging
National Institute on Deafness and Other Communication Disorders
Sound World Solutions

Hearing Loop System provided by Contacta, Inc.

Workshop Objectives

- Describe and characterize the public health significance of hearing loss and the relationship between hearing loss and healthy aging.
- Examine and explore current and future areas of research.
- Discuss comprehensive hearing rehabilitative strategies, including innovative models of care.
- Explore innovative hearing technologies and barriers to their development and use.
- Consider and discuss short- and long-term collaborative strategies for approaching age-related hearing loss as a public health priority.

DAY ONE: January 13, 2014

9:00 a.m.   **Welcome and Opening Remarks**
                Alan M. Jette, *Workshop Co-Chair*
                Boston University School of Public Health

                Frank R. Lin, *Workshop Co-Chair*
                Johns Hopkins University

CONSUMER PERSPECTIVE ON THE IMPACT OF HEARING LOSS

9:30 a.m.   Katherine Bouton, Author, *Shouting Won't Help*

SESSION I: AGING AND HEARING LOSS: WHY DOES IT MATTER?

9:50 a.m.   **Introductions**
                Frank R. Lin *(Moderator)*
                Johns Hopkins University

9:55 a.m.   **Series of Presentations**
                Luigi Ferrucci, National Institute on Aging
                James Firman, National Council on Aging
                Kathleen Pichora-Fuller, University of Toronto

10:25 a.m.   **Discussion with Speakers and Audience**

SESSION II: THE CONNECTION BETWEEN HEARING LOSS AND HEALTHY AGING

10:45 a.m.   **Introductions**
                Luigi Ferrucci *(Moderator)*
                National Institute on Aging

10:50 a.m.   Series of Presentations

Impact on Cognition
Marilyn Albert, Johns Hopkins University School of
    Medicine

Impact on Physical Functioning
Alan M. Jette, Boston University School of Public Health

Psychosocial Impacts
Barbara Weinstein, Graduate School and University
    Center, City University of New York

11:40 a.m.   Discussion with Speakers and Audience

**SESSION III: CURRENT APPROACHES TO
HEARING HEALTH CARE DELIVERY**

1:15 p.m.   Introductions
Lucille B. Beck *(Moderator)*
U.S. Department of Veterans Affairs

1:20 p.m.   Series of Presentations

The Spectrum of Hearing Impairment
Theresa Hnath Chisolm, University of South Florida

The Current U.S. Hearing Health Model
Margaret I. Wallhagen, University of California,
    San Francisco

International Perspective
Nikolai Bisgaard, GN ReSound A/S

2:35 p.m.   Discussion with Speakers and Audience

SESSION IV: INNOVATIVE MODELS

3:30 p.m.   Introductions
Nikolai Bisgaard *(Moderator)*
GN ReSound A/S

3:35 p.m.   Series of Presentations

                   Community Health Workers[1]
                   Nicole Marrone, University of Arizona

                   Teleaudiology
                   Gabrielle Saunders, Portland VA Medical Center

                   *Addressing Untreated Age-Related Hearing Loss in a
                   Primary Care Setting*
                   Thomas Powers, Powers Family Practice

4:20 p.m.   **Discussion with Speakers and Audience**

4:50 p.m.   **Day 1 Reflections and Closing Remarks**

5:00 p.m.   **Adjourn Day 1**

                   DAY TWO: January 14, 2014

9:00 a.m.   Welcome
                   Alan M. Jette, *Workshop Co-Chair*
                   Boston University School of Public Health

                   Frank R. Lin, *Workshop Co-Chair*
                   Johns Hopkins University

                   SESSION V: HEARING TECHNOLOGIES

9:05 a.m.   Introductions
                   Brenda Battat *(Moderator)*
                   Hearing Loss Association of America (Retired)

9:10 a.m.   Series of Presentations

                   Technology Overview
                   Cynthia Compton-Conley, Compton-Conley Consulting

---

[1] This presentation was prepared by Nicole Marrone, assistant professor and James S. and Dyan Pignatelli/Unisource Clinical Chair in Audiologic Rehabilitation for Adults at the University of Arizona, but due to unforeseen circumstances, was presented by Theresa Chisolm.

FDA Regulation of Hearing Aids
Eric A. Mann, U.S. Food and Drug Administration

Technology Assessment
Fiona Miller, University of Toronto

10:10 a.m.   Discussion with Speakers and Audience

HEARING TECHNOLOGIES FROM A CONSUMER PERSPECTIVE

10:55 a.m.   Richard Einhorn, Composer, *Voices of Light*

SESSION VI: AGING AND HEARING LOSS: WHY DOES IT MATTER?

11:15 a.m.   Introductions
Karen J. Cruickshanks *(Moderator)*
University of Wisconsin School of Medicine and
    Public Health

11:20 a.m.   Series of Presentations

Lessons in Innovation
David Green, Sound World Solutions

The Function and Importance of Wireless Standards
Stephen Berger, TEM Consulting

Universal Design
Valerie Fletcher, Institute for Human Centered Design

12:20 p.m.   Discussion with Speakers and Audience

SESSION VII: CONTEMPORARY ISSUES IN HEARING HEALTH CARE

1:45 p.m.   Introductions
Carole M. Rogin *(Moderator)*
Hearing Industries Association

1:50 p.m.   Series of Presentations

                   Healthy People 2001–2020: Tracking Age-Related
                   Measures of Hearing Health in the New Millennium
                   Howard J. Hoffman, National Institute on Deafness
                       and Other Communication Disorders, National
                       Institutes of Health (NIDCD/NIH)

                   The Changing Hearing Healthcare Landscape
                   Robert Burkard, University at Buffalo

                   NIDCD Research Working Group on Accessible and
                   Affordable Hearing Health Care
                   Amy M. Donahue, National Institute on Deafness and
                       Other Communication Disorders, National Institutes
                       of Health (NIDCD/NIH)
                   Judy R. Dubno, Medical University of South Carolina
                   Lucille B. Beck, U.S. Department of Veterans Affairs

2:35 p.m.   Discussion with Speakers and Audience

SESSION VIII: COLLABORATIVE STRATEGIES FOR THE FUTURE

3:05 p.m.   Reactions and Discussion
                   James Firman *(Moderator)*, National Council on Aging
                   Regina Davis Moss, American Public Health Association
                   James Pacala, American Geriatrics Society and University
                       of Minnesota Medical School
                   Charlotte Yeh, AARP

3:40 p.m.   Discussion with Speakers and Audience

4:05 p.m.   Closing Remarks
                   Alan M. Jette, *Workshop Co-Chair*
                   Boston University School of Public Health

                   Frank R. Lin, *Workshop Co-Cchair*
                   Johns Hopkins University

4:20 p.m.   Adjourn

Appendix B

Speaker Biographical Sketches

Marilyn Albert, Ph.D., is professor of neurology and the director of the Division of Cognitive Neuroscience in the Department of Neurology at Johns Hopkins University School of Medicine. She is also the director of the Johns Hopkins Alzheimer's Disease Research Center. Her major research interests are in the area of cognitive change with age, and disease-related changes of cognition (with a particular focus on the early diagnosis of Alzheimer's disease). Her research has focused on the relationship of cognitive change to brain structure and function, as assessed through imaging and other biomarkers. She has written more than 200 peer-reviewed publications.

Brenda Battat, M.S., is the retired executive director of the Hearing Loss Association of America (HLAA). During 24 years with the HLAA, 5 as executive director, she led nationwide advocacy efforts to change the way society views hearing loss, pushed for accessible and affordable hearing health care and consumer choice in the marketplace, promoted hearing-friendly environments through technology such as looping and captioning, and successfully advocated for hearing-aid-compatible mobile products. She upheld the philosophy of self-help and encouraged and taught consumers to self-advocate. Ms. Battat has served on government, professional, and business advisory boards, including the U.S. Access Board's Telecommunications Access Advisory Committee, the Federal Communications Commission's Consumer/Disability Advisory Committee, the AT&T Advisory Panel on Access and Aging, the National Advisory Group—National Technical Institute for the Deaf, the American and Northwest Airlines Consumer Advisory Committees, and the National Institute on Deafness and Other

Communication Disorders (NIDCD) Advisory Council of the National Institutes of Health (NIH). Ms. Battat received an M.S. in education from Indiana University and B.Sc. in physical therapy from St. Mary's Hospital, London, England. For her work she received the Sheldon Williams Itzkoff Leadership Award (2010); Robert H. Weitbrecht Telecommunications Access Award (2007); Oticon Focus on People Advocacy Award (2005); and Self Help for Hard of Hearing People National Access Award (2002).

Lucille B. Beck, Ph.D., is chief consultant, Rehabilitation and Prosthetic Services, as well as director of the Audiology and Speech Pathology Program in the Office of Patient Care Services, Veterans Health Administration for the Department of Veterans Affairs (VA). She is also chief of Audiology and Speech Pathology Service at the Washington, DC, VA Medical Center. As chief consultant for Rehabilitation and Prosthetic Services, her responsibilities include oversight and direction for Audiology and Speech Pathology Service, Blind Rehabilitation Service, Physical Medicine and Rehabilitation Service and Polytrauma, Recreation Therapy Service, and Prosthetic and Sensory Aids Service. Dr. Beck received the Presidential Rank Award for Meritorious Executive Service in 2000, and in 2007 she received the Presidential Rank Award for Distinguished Executive Service. The Pennsylvania College of Optometry School of Audiology conferred an honorary doctor of science degree on Dr. Beck in 2008 for her commitment to Americans with hearing loss. Dr. Beck received her Ph.D. from the University of Maryland. She has jointly held faculty appointments at Gallaudet University, George Washington University, and the University of Maryland. She has authored numerous publications and scientific papers and is a well-known presenter on topics ranging from amplification, outcomes, patient satisfaction, professional issues in audiology, and rehabilitation for the nation's veterans. She is a recognized expert in hearing technology.

Stephen Berger is president of TEM Consulting, an engineering services and consulting firm in Austin, Texas. Mr. Berger has an extensive background in standards development. He has served on three federal advisory committees, two of which were charged with issues related to disability access. He has chaired five standards that have been adopted by the Federal Communications Commission into the Code of Federal Regulations. He has also been president of the International Association of Radio and Telecommunications Engineers.

Nikolai Bisgaard, M.Sc., serves as vice president of Intellectual Property Rights and industry relations at GN ReSound A/S. He has worked for GN ReSound since 1978 and served as vice president of research and development there for 15 years. He has been a director at GN Store Nord A/S since

2006. He currently manages the intellectual property rights function at GN ReSound while also spending significant time on hearing industry politics and professional issues related to hearing aid use, including responsibility for the biannual International Symposium on Auditory and Audiological Research sponsored by GN ReSound. He is also cochair of the scientific program for Nordic Audiology College. Mr. Bisgaard has been active in the European Hearing Instrument Manufacturers Association (EHIMA) for decades and is currently chairman of the Market Development Committee, where initiatives for informing the public on hearing matters as well as consumer research are managed. From 2007 to 2010 he was a major contributor to the European Committee for Standardization (CEN) 15927 standard for services offered by hearing aid professionals. He is the author of many scientific articles ranging from clinical testing of feedback suppression systems to standard audiograms for hearing aid characterization. He holds an M.Sc. in electrical engineering from the Technical University of Denmark, where he mastered in psychoacoustics.

Katherine Bouton is the author of *Shouting Won't Help,* a memoir of adult-onset hearing loss published in 2013 by Sarah Crichton/Farrar Straus and Giroux. She is a former editor at the *New York Times*, where she was deputy editor of the Sunday magazine for 10 years. She also held senior editing positions for *Science Times*, the *Sunday Book Review*, and *Culture*. She is at work on a second book on hearing loss, tentatively titled *Come to Your Senses: Learn to Live Better with Hearing Loss.* She has had progressive bilateral hearing loss since 1978 and in September 2009 received a cochlear implant. Her writing and speaking now focus on hearing loss and other disability issues. She is a graduate of Vassar College and is a member of the board of trustees of the HLAA.

Robert Burkard, Ph.D., CCC-A, is professor and chair in the Department of Rehabilitation Science, University at Buffalo. His research interests have included acoustic calibration, auditory electrophysiology (in particular, auditory evoked potentials), vestibular/balance function/dysfunction, functional imaging, and aging. His professional interests currently involve acoustical standards and health care economics.

Theresa (Terry) Hnath Chisolm, Ph.D., CCC-A, completed her undergraduate degree at Lehman College, her master's degree in audiology at Montclair State College, and her Ph.D. in speech and hearing sciences at the Graduate School of the City University of New York (CUNY). She joined the faculty in the Department of Communication Sciences and Disorders at the University of South Florida as an assistant professor in 1988. She is currently a full professor and department chair, having served as chair since 2004. Her area of research and clinical expertise is rehabilitative audiology in children and adults. She has received funding for her research from the NIDCD/ NIH, VA Merit Reviews, and contracts with the hearing aid industry. Dr. Chisolm currently is co-principal investigator on a U.S. Department of Education Office of Special Education Programs grant for training master's degree students in speech-language pathology to work with children with hearing loss who come from culturally diverse backgrounds from a listening and spoken language perspective. In 2011 Dr. Chisolm received the Distinguished Achievement Award from the American Academy of Audiology.

Cynthia Compton-Conley, Ph.D., has enjoyed a distinguished career as an audiologist, educator, consultant, and consumer advocate. Her in-depth knowledge of assistive technologies for providing receptive communication access has made her a popular public speaker. Dr. Compton-Conley developed a proven systems engineering approach to hearing enhancement that skillfully integrates needs assessment, technology insertion, and related training to provide receptive communication access tailored to each individual's lifestyle and hearing challenges at home, in the workplace, and in other relevant venues. An alumnus of Rutgers University, Vanderbilt University, and CUNY, Dr. Compton-Conley taught doctoral students in audiology for many years at Gallaudet University, where she also served as founder and director of the Gallaudet Assistive Devices Center. She has been the recipient of many honors and awards, including the Special Friends of Hearing Impaired People Award from the Hearing Loss Association and the Distinguished Achievement Award from the American Academy of Audiology. Following her teaching career, she served, for 2 years, as director of hearing wellness at Etymotic Research, where she developed a website, www.soundstrategy.com, that serves as a resource for individuals seeking guidance on hearing enhancement techniques. Currently, she is the chief executive officer (CEO) of Compton-Conley Consulting, whose services include (1) hearing enhancement coaching to individuals, providers, corporations, and government agencies, (2) ADA compliance training and expert witness services, (3) consulting to industry and working groups who are leveraging leading-edge/bleeding-edge technologies toward hearing enhancement solutions, and (4) providing website/blogosphere content associated with hearing wellness, needs assessment, and new technology.

Karen J. Cruickshanks, Ph.D., completed her Ph.D. in epidemiology at the University of Pittsburgh Graduate School of Public Health in 1987 and has been a faculty member at the University of Wisconsin–Madison since 1990. Her research program is studying the health problems of aging through epidemiological cohort studies. The Epidemiology of Hearing Loss Study

(EHLS) is funded by the National Institute on Aging (NIA) (AG11099) to study hearing, olfactory, and cognitive impairments in a population-based cohort of 3,500 older residents of Beaver Dam, Wisconsin. The focus of this research is on the roles of inflammation and vascular factors on age-related disorders. In 2004, a new study of the adult offspring of the EHLS participants was funded by the NIA, National Eye Institute, and NIDCD (AG021917) to study the genetic and environmental factors that contribute to age-related sensory impairments. She was the principal investigator of the EpiSense Audiometry Reading Center for the Hispanic Community Health Study, a multicenter study including hearing testing for 16,000 Latinos. A major theme of her research is the link between subclinical atherosclerosis and the sensory and neurological disorders of aging.

Regina Davis Moss, Ph.D., M.P.H., MCHES, is the associate executive director of public health policy and practice for the American Public Health Association, where she oversees a broad portfolio of programs and activities ranging from continuing education to global health. She has nearly 20 years of experience managing national health promotion and disease prevention initiatives addressing such areas as reproductive health, healthy aging, obesity prevention, health policy, and sustained capacity in public health. Formerly, Dr. Davis Moss held a senior management position for a healthy eating and active living education effort for the federal government. Prior to that, she worked for the Henry J. Kaiser Family Foundation (KFF), where she helped launched the Kaiser Health News online information service and served as the senior producer. Dr. Davis Moss came to KFF after serving as a supervisor for one of the first U.S. research studies to investigate the prevalence of uterine fibroid tumors. She also served as a public health service fellow in the Office on Women's Health for the U.S. Department of Health and Human Services. Dr. Davis Moss is a master certified health education specialist; a member of the Delta Omega Honorary Public Health Society; and author of several journal articles and reports focusing on gestational weight gain, health communications, and family health policy. She is a member of the executive board of the National Healthy Start Association, the Ad Council's Advisory Committee on Public Issues, and an appointed member of the District of Columbia Mayor's Council on Physical Fitness, Health and Nutrition. Dr. Davis Moss earned a doctorate of philosophy in maternal and child health from the University of Maryland, College Park, a master's degree in public health from George Washington University, a B.S. in biology from Howard University, and a public health certificate in performance improvement from the University of Minnesota. Her professional areas of interest include women's reproductive health, adolescent health, and health equity.

Amy M. Donahue, Ph.D., presently serves as deputy director, Division of Scientific Programs, and coordinator of the Hearing and Balance/Vestibular Sciences Program at the NIDCD/NIH. She is responsible for overseeing the program planning, coordination, and conduct of grant research in hearing and balance/vestibular sciences. She has been at the NIDCD since 1991 and has been responsible for the creation of numerous scientific initiatives in hearing and balance sciences. Many of her activities have been instrumental in increasing NIDCD support for translational research, clinical research, and patient-oriented outcomes research activities. Dr. Donahue received her master's degree in audiology (1979) and her Ph.D. in speech and hearing science (1985) from the University of Tennessee, Knoxville. She is a member of several professional organizations, has numerous professional publications and presentations, has served on various organizational and technical committees, and has received awards of recognition. Dr. Donahue has cultivated collaborative relationships with the extramural research community, professional organizations, and numerous federal agency partners.

Judy R. Dubno, Ph.D., is a professor in the Department of Otolaryngology–Head and Neck Surgery at the Medical University of South Carolina in Charleston. Her research, which is supported by grants from the NIDCD/NIH, focuses on auditory perception and speech recognition in adverse listening conditions and how perception changes with age, hearing loss, hearing aids, and training. She served on the NIDCD Advisory Council of the NIH, as president of the Association for Research in Otolaryngology, and is currently president-elect of the Acoustical Society of America. She is a Fellow of the Acoustical Society of America and the American Speech-Language-Hearing Association and the recipient of the James Jerger Career Award for Research in Audiology.

Richard Einhorn is a critically acclaimed composer and classical record producer. Since losing much of his hearing overnight in 2010, he has used his lifelong knowledge of audio technology to hear better in situations where hearing aids are inadequate. He has also become a well-known advocate for improved assistive listening technologies. His advocacy for public use of induction loop systems and his innovative use of an iPhone to hear better in noisy restaurants have been featured on NPR and in numerous articles in the *New York Times, Washington Post, Business Week*, and other major media. On February 22, 2014, Mr. Einhorn's oratorio with silent film, *Voices of Light*, was performed at the National Cathedral of Washington.

Luigi Ferrucci, M.D., Ph.D., is a geriatrician and epidemiologist who conducts research on the causal pathways leading to progressive physical and cognitive decline in older persons. In September 2002, he became the chief of the Longitudinal Studies Section at NIA and the director of the Baltimore Longitudinal Study on Aging. Dr. Ferrucci received a medical degree and board certification in 1980, a board certification in geriatrics in 1982, and Ph.D. in biology and pathophysiology of aging in 1998 at the University of Florence, Italy. He spent many years as associate professor of biology, human physiology, and statistics at the University of Florence. Between 1985 and 2002 he was chief of geriatric rehabilitation at the Department of Geriatric Medicine and director of the Laboratory of Clinical Epidemiology at the Italian National Institute of Aging. During the same period, he collaborated with the NIA Laboratory of Epidemiology, Demography, and Biometry, where he spent several periods as visiting scientist. Dr. Ferrucci has made major contributions in the design of many epidemiological studies conducted in the United States and in Europe, including the European Longitudinal Study on Aging, the "ICare Dicomano Study," the AKEA study of Centenarians in Sardinia, and the Women's Health and Aging Study. He was also the principal investigator of the InCHIANTI study, a longitudinal study conducted in the Chianti geographical area (Tuscany, Italy), looking at risk factors for mobility disability in older persons. Dr. Ferrucci has redesigned the Baltimore Longitudinal Study on Aging to retain the wealth of data collected over more than 50 years while introducing new questions on the nature of aging that have emerged in the recent literature. Dr. Ferrucci is scientific director, NIA, since May 2011.

James Firman, Ed.D., M.B.A., has been the president and CEO of the National Council on Aging (NCOA) since 1995. Under his leadership, NCOA has developed many nationally acclaimed programs to improve the health, independence, and continuing contributions of older adults. Firman has also served in several leadership roles in the field of aging, including chair of the Leadership Council of Aging Organizations (twice), chair of the Access to Benefits Coalition, and board member of Generations United and the National Human Services Assembly. Prior to joining NCOA as president and CEO, Firman was president and CEO of the United Seniors Health Cooperative (USHC), a nonprofit consumer organization, for 10 years. At the USHC, he directed the development of the nation's first line-of-credit reverse mortgages; the Cooperative Caring Network, a major community-wide volunteer service-credit program that helps frail and disabled persons remain at home; and early generations of benefits screening software. From 1981 to 1984, Firman served as a senior program officer at the Robert Wood Johnson Foundation, where he helped develop initiatives in aging and health care finance, as well as the model Interfaith Volunteer Caregivers program. He is a cofounder of Grantmakers in Aging. Firman is a noted expert and consumer advocate on many issues affecting older persons, including public policy, long-term care, health insurance, finance issues, and

intergenerational programs. He has provided expert testimony before many
congressional committees. He has written several books and many articles
on issues in aging, for consumers as well as professionals. Dr. Firman holds
a master's degree in business administration and a doctorate in education
from Columbia University.

Valerie Fletcher has been executive director since 1998 of the Boston-based
Institute for Human Centered Design, an international educational and
design nonprofit organization founded in 1978. The organizational mission
is to advance the role of design in expanding opportunity and enhancing
experience for people of all ages and abilities through excellence in design.
Ms. Fletcher writes, lectures, and works internationally. Her research focus is engaging user/experts in analysis of the usability in places and in
products. She is a special advisor on inclusive design to the Open Society
Institute, the governments of France and Singapore, and the UN Department of Economic and Social Affairs. Ms. Fletcher has a master's degree
in ethics and public policy from Harvard University. The Boston Society of
Architects awarded her the Women in Design award in 2005. She cochairs
the Design Industry Group of Massachusetts and is a founding member of
the International Association for Universal Design in Tokyo.

David Green, M.P.H., has worked with many organizations to make medical technology and health care services sustainable, affordable, and accessible to all. Mr. Green is a MacArthur Fellow and an Ashoka Fellow
and has been recognized by the Schwab Foundation as a leading social
entrepreneur. Mr. Green directed the establishment of Aurolab (India) to
produce affordable intraocular lenses (now with 10 percent of the global
market share), suture, and pharmaceuticals. He has developed high-volume,
quality eye care programs that are affordable and self-sustaining from user
fees. At Aravind Eye Hospital in India, which performs more than 370,000
surgeries per year, 50 percent of the care is provided free of charge or below cost, yet the hospital is able to generate substantial surplus revenue.
He has helped to develop major eye care programs in Bangladesh, China,
Egypt, Guatemala, India, Nepal, and Tanzania. Within this paradigm of
"empathetic capitalism," he now works to create social investing funds to
support sustainable social enterprises (The Eye Fund with Deutsche Bank
for $15M). He cofounded Sound World Solutions, a social enterprise to
make affordable hearing devices with a novel fitting, and Brien Holden
Vision Diagnostics to design unique and affordable ways to detect eye
disease, diabetes, and neurological disorders. He works with the Pacific
Vision Foundation to establish an eye institute serving all people in north-
ern California. Mr. Green is also vice president at Ashoka, where he leads
an effort to reduce health care costs in the United States. He graduated

from the University of Michigan with a bachelor's degree in general studies (1978) and a master's degree in public health (1982). He is on the faculty of Johns Hopkins Wilmer Eye Institute. He is the recipient of the 2009 Spirit of Helen Keller award for humanitarian efforts in blindness prevention; is the recipient of the 2009 University of Michigan Humanitarian Service Award; and was selected by University of Michigan engineering students as a leading social entrepreneur alumnus. He is on the boards of the University of Michigan School of Business Social Venture Fund and the Stanford Biomedical Fellowship for India and is on the advisory board of the Seva Foundation.

Howard J. Hoffman, M.A., is director, Epidemiology and Statistics Program, NIDCD/NIH. Since 1992, he has led this research program, which focuses on the prevalence, incidence, risk factors, and preventive interventions for conditions or disorders of NIDCD's seven mission areas: hearing, balance, smell, taste, voice, speech, and language. He has published more than 200 peer-reviewed biomedical/scientific articles, written several book chapters, and edited 2 books. He has served as NIDCD project officer for the National Health and Nutrition Examination Survey (NHANES) Hearing, Balance, and Chemosensory components and for other epidemiologic studies (for example, the 2008 National Health Interview Survey [NHIS] Dizziness and Balance Supplement and the 2012 NHIS Voice, Speech and Language Supplement). He was NIDCD lead coordinator for the 8 hearing health objectives in *Healthy People 2010* and continues in this role for *Healthy People 2020*, which was expanded to include 23 objectives embracing all 7 of the institute's mission areas.

Alan M. Jette, Ph.D., M.P.H., currently directs Boston University's Health and Disability Research Institute. From 1996 to 2004 he served as professor and dean of Boston University's Sargent College of Health and Rehabilitation Sciences. Dr. Jette currently serves as research director for the New England Regional Spinal Cord Injury Center based at Boston University Medical Center and as associate director of the Boston Claude Pepper Center on Aging Research. Dr. Jette currently directs the Boston Rehabilitation Outcomes Measurement Center, funded by the NIH National Center for Medical Rehabilitation Research. He received a B.S. in physical therapy from the State University of New York at Buffalo in 1973 and his M.P.H. (1975) and Ph.D. (1979) in public health from the University of Michigan.

Frank R. Lin, M.D., Ph.D., is an assistant professor of otolaryngology, geriatric medicine, mental health, and epidemiology at the Johns Hopkins University School of Medicine and the Bloomberg School of Public Health. Dr. Lin completed his medical education, residency in otolaryngology, and

Ph.D. in clinical investigation at Johns Hopkins. He completed further oto-
logic fellowship training in Lucerne, Switzerland. Dr. Lin's clinical practice
is dedicated to otology and the medical and surgical management of hearing
loss. His epidemiologic research focuses on how hearing loss impacts the
health and functioning of older adults and the role of hearing rehabilitative
strategies in potentially mitigating these effects. In particular, his research
group has demonstrated that hearing loss in older adults is strongly and independently associated with the risk of cognitive decline, incident dementia,
impairments in physical functioning and mobility, and greater health care
resource utilization. He collaborates extensively with researchers across
multiple fields, including gerontology, cognitive neuroscience, audiology,
and epidemiology, and he has collaborative working relationships with
individuals in industry, government, and nonprofit advocacy organizations.
His research has been extensively covered in the media, including the *New
York Times* and the BBC, and he has appeared on CBS *This Morning* and
the *Charlie Rose* show.

Eric A. Mann, M.D., Ph.D., CAPT, USPHS, serves as the clinical deputy
director for the Division of Ophthalmic and Ear, Nose, and Throat Devices in the Center for Devices and Radiological Health (CDRH) at the
U.S. Food and Drug Administration. He earned his M.D. and his Ph.D. in
microbiology and immunology from the Medical College of Pennsylvania
in 1988. After his internship in general surgery at St. Francis Hospital
and Medical Center, Hartford, Connecticut, he completed a residency in
otolaryngology–head and neck surgery at the University of Connecticut
Health Center, Farmington, in 1993. He is board certified in his specialty
and previously served as attending surgeon at the Walter Reed Army Medical Center (1993–1997) in Washingon, DC, and as senior staff surgeon at
the NIH Clinical Center in Bethesda, Maryland (1999–2001). He holds an
appointment as assistant professor of surgery at the Uniformed Services
University of the Health Sciences in Bethesda and serves as a commissioned
officer in the U.S. Public Health Service. He has been actively involved in
the premarket regulation of devices since his arrival at CDRH in 2001.

Nicole Marrone, Ph.D., CCC-A, holds the James S. and Dyan Pignatelli/
Unisource Clinical Chair in Audiologic Rehabilitation for Adults at the
University of Arizona and is an assistant professor in the Department of
Speech, Language, and Hearing Sciences. Her research investigates hearing
loss and rehabilitation in adults. She is currently collaborating with public
health researchers and community health workers to increase access to
hearing healthcare among older adults on the U.S.-Mexico border. This
interdisciplinary research is supported by the NIH.

Fiona Miller, Ph.D., is an associate professor of health policy in the Institute of Health Policy, Management and Evaluation, and she heads the Division of Health Policy and Ethics at the Toronto Health Economics and Technology Assessment (THETA) Collaborative at the University of Toronto. Her program of research centers on health technology policy, including the dynamics of health technology development, assessment, and adoption within systems of health research and health care.

James Pacala, M.D., M.S., a board-certified family physician and geriatrician, is Distinguished Teaching Professor and associate head, Department of Family Medicine and Community Health at the University of Minnesota Medical School. Dr. Pacala is board chair of the American Geriatrics Society (AGS). He has performed research and published extensively on models of care delivery to geriatric populations and on innovative teaching methods. In addition, Dr. Pacala has served as co-author of the AGS practice handbook *Geriatrics at Your Fingertips*, now in its 15th edition, with more than 250,000 copies sold. Dr. Pacala was co-editor-in-chief of the AGS's comprehensive geriatrics resource, the *Geriatrics Review Syllabus* (7th edition), published in 2010. He is extensively involved in medical student education nationally and at the University of Minnesota Medical School. Dr. Pacala has received several awards for his research, teaching, and clinical care, including AGS's Outstanding Achievement for Clinical Investigation Award (2002), the University of Minnesota Medical School's Outstanding Teacher of the Year Award (1999), the University of Minnesota's All-University Postbaccalaureate, Graduate, and Professional Education Teaching Award (2002), and the University of Minnesota Academic Health Center Award for Excellence in the Scholarship of Teaching (2009). He received his baccalaureate degree from Carleton College and his M.D. from the University of Rochester School of Medicine and Dentistry. After completing a residency in family medicine at the University of Wisconsin–Madison, Dr. Pacala obtained a master's degree in chronic disease epidemiology from Brown University and completed two fellowships, one in health services research in gerontology (at Brown University) and the other in clinical geriatrics (at the University of Connecticut). He has been on the faculty at the University of Minnesota since 1992.

Kathleen Pichora-Fuller, Ph.D., is a full professor of psychology at the University of Toronto Mississauga. She is also an adjunct scientist at the Toronto Rehabilitation Institute and at the Rotman Research Institute at Baycrest and is a guest professor at the Linneaus Centre for Hearing and Deafness Research at Linköping University in Sweden. She completed a B.A. in linguistics at the University of Toronto (1977) and a M.Sc. in audiology and speech sciences at the University of British Columbia (1980).

She worked as a clinical audiologist and then the supervisor of audiology at Mount Sinai Hospital in Toronto, and then she returned to complete a Ph.D. in psychology at the University of Toronto (1991). Until 2002, she was a faculty member in the faculty of medicine and director of the Institute for Hearing Accessibility Research at the University of British Columbia. Her research is funded by the Natural Sciences and Engineering Research Council of Canada and the Canadian Institutes of Health Research, and she is the hearing expert for the Canadian Longitudinal Study of Aging. She is now translating her lab-based research to address the needs of older adults who suffer from both hearing and cognitive impairments. She was president of the Canadian Association of Speech Language Pathologists and Audiologists (1984–1987) and served on the executive boards of the Canadian Acoustical Association (1998–2002, 2011–present), the International Collegium of Rehabilitative Audiology (1997–2003), and the Canadian Academy of Audiology (2002–2004). She was also the Canadian representative to the International Society of Audiology (2004–2010). She is presently on the editorial boards of two international journals.

Thomas Powers, M.D., is a Fellow of the American Academy of Family Physicians. Dr. Powers has been a solo practioner for 25 years in Lake Havasu City, Arizona.

Carole Rogin, M.A., is a speech-language pathologist by training. She worked as a sleep-language pathologist for 5 years and then joined the staff at the American Speech-Language-Hearing Association. Ms. Rogin joined the Hearing Industries Association as its first director of market development in 1980. Since that time she has served not only as the director of market development but also as the president and executive director of the association. Her role has been working to bring the industry together to strengthen the ties between the manufacturers and the dispensing and consumer communities.

Gabrielle Saunders, Ph.D., is associate director of the VA Rehabilitation Research and Development National Center for Rehabilitative Auditory Research (NCRAR), Portland VA Medical Center, Portland, Oregon, and associate professor in the Department of Otolaryngology at Oregon Health and Science University, also in Portland. Over the past 20 years, Dr. Saunders's research program has worked to optimize outcomes of auditory rehabilitation by furthering the understanding of hearing-related behaviors and individual differences that impact outcomes. To this end, she has made contributions to the field through the development of questionnaires and educational and counseling interventions. Her work focuses on understanding and changing hearing-related behaviors, optimizing hearing rehabilitation outcomes, and researching how to prevent hearing loss. She has several ongoing funded research studies, including work examining hearing health care behaviors of help seeking, the use of auditory rehabilitation and hearing conservation from the perspective of health behavior theory, the application of principles of adult learning theory and a universal approach to health literacy to improve delivery of information to patients during clinical encounters, and the examination of interventions for auditory rehabilitation to obtain an evidence base for their effectiveness. In addition to her research endeavors, Dr. Saunders oversees student mentoring and training programs at the NCRAR, chairs the biennial NCRAR conferences, and directs other NCRAR education and outreach programs.

Margaret I. Wallhagen, Ph.D., GNP-BC, AGSF, FAAN, is a professor of gerontological nursing and a geriatric nurse practitioner in the School of Nursing, University of California, San Francisco (UCSF). She received her initial nursing degree from St. Luke's Hospital School of Nursing in New York, her baccalaureate and master's degrees from UCSF, and her doctoral degree in nursing from the University of Washington in Seattle. Her prior clinical nursing experience has included critical care nursing and precepting undergraduate nursing students. Since joining the faculty at UCSF in 1988, she has taught gerontological nursing at both the masters and doctoral level, and works as a Geriatric Nurse Practitioner. Dr. Wallhagen has conducted a number of research projects in gerontology and chronic care management. Her research and publications focus on studies of the experience of control in caregivers and in persons with diabetes; education and self-management in diabetes; successful aging for persons with chronic conditions; self-care and symptom management; cross-cultural interventions to support family caregivers with dementia; family conflict and coping; and the impact of hearing impairment on older adults. Her research and publications have focused on the areas of informal caregiving, the experience of control, successful aging and diabetes, but with a major focus for over a decade on the impact of hearing impairment on older adults and their families. She recently completed a 4-year longitudinal study of the experience of hearing impairment in older adults and their partners and is currently working on a project that is testing an intervention to embed hearing screening and education into primary care settings. In January 2006, Dr. Wallhagen became the director of the UCSF/John A. Hartford Center of Geriatric Nursing Excellence as it entered its second 5 years of funding. This center's mission is to prepare a cadre of nurses who have the research, leadership, and educational expertise necessary to facilitate the preparation of future nurse leaders and to meet the needs of the growing population of older adults. Most recently, Dr. Wallhagen became the senior nurse faculty mentor for the Veterans Affairs National Quality Scholars Fellowship Program, a program designed to prepare participants to develop and apply new knowledge for the ongoing improvement of health care services for the VA and the nation. In addition to her teaching and research work, Dr. Wallhagen has been involved with and has served on the board of the Family Caregiver Alliance, a nonprofit organization that supports family caregivers, and Bread for the World, an organization that works for policies to eliminate hunger worldwide. Over the past several years she has worked with the Hearing Loss Association of America. She is currently on the board of trustees of the association and is committed to facilitating the achievement of its mission.

Barbara Weinstein, Ph.D., is a professor of audiology and speech language hearing sciences and the founding executive officer of the health sciences doctoral programs and the Au.D. program at the Graduate School and University Center, CUNY. Dr. Weinstein earned her Ph.D. in audiology at Columbia University, having written her dissertation on social isolation and hearing loss in the elderly. The focus of her research has been on documenting and quantifying the psychosocial effects of hearing loss in older adults, quantifying the psychosocial effects of hearing loss, determining the epidemiology of hearing loss in older adults, and performing outcomes assessment. More recently, she has transitioned to promoting patient-centered care among older adults with hearing loss and educating primary care physicians regarding identification of older adults with hearing loss. Dr. Weinstein is the author of *Geriatric Audiology*, volumes 1 and 2. She is the co-developer of the Hearing Handicap Inventory for the Elderly and for Adults, a self-report scale used globally to quantify the functional effects of hearing loss on older adults and family members. The recipient of numerous awards for her contribution to the understanding of the psychosocial effects of hearing loss on older adults, Dr. Weinstein is the author of more than 75 manuscripts on hearing loss in older adults.

Charlotte Yeh, M.D., FACEP, is the chief medical officer for AARP Services, Inc. She is responsible for working with AARP's health carriers on programs that lead to enhanced care for older adults. Dr. Yeh has more than 30 years of health care experience—as a practitioner of emergency medicine at Newton-Wellesley Hospital and Tufts Medical Center, as the medical director for the National Heritage Insurance Company, as a Medicare Part B claims contractor, and as the regional administrator at the Centers for Medicare & Medicaid Services in Boston. Dr. Yeh is widely recognized for her commitment to and passion for the health care consumer and has received numerous honors for her efforts on behalf of patients. Dr. Yeh received a B.A. from Northwestern University and her medical degree from Northwestern University Medical School. She completed her internship in general surgery at the University of Washington and her residency in emergency medicine at the University of California, Los Angeles.